Good Clean Food

Good Clean Food

Shopping Smart to Avoid GMOs, rBGH, and Products That May Cause Cancer and Other Diseases

By Samuel Epstein, MD, and Beth Leibson

Foreword by Gary Null, PhD

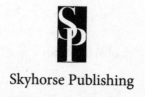

Skyhorse Publishing

Skyhorse Publishing books may be purchased in bulk at special discounts for sales promotion, corporate gifts, fund-raising, or educational purposes. Special editions can also be created to specifications. For details, contact the Special Sales Department, Skyhorse Publishing, 307 West 36th Street, 11th Floor, New York, NY 10018 or info@skyhorsepublishing.com.

Skyhorse® and Skyhorse Publishing® are registered trademarks of Skyhorse Publishing, Inc.®, a Delaware corporation.

Visit our website at www.skyhorsepublishing.com.

10 9 8 7 6 5 4 3 2 1

Library of Congress Cataloging-in-Publication Data is available on file.
ISBN: 978-1-61608-821-7

Printed in the United States of America

Contents

Foreword

by Gary Null, PhD

Author of *The Complete Encyclopedia of Natural Healing* and host of
The Gary Null Show

In *Good Clean Food*, Dr. Samuel Epstein, one of our most insightful and authoritative voices on avoidable causes of cancer, has teamed up with health writer Beth Leibson to once again present persuasive and well-documented evidence on the hidden health risks of everyday consumer products.

Good Clean Food does more than educate us as to the importance of avoiding industrial carcinogens in our food; it also presents scientific evidence compelling us to do so. Although warnings about the nation's crisis in unsafe foods are continually mounting, the Food and Drug Administration continues to disregard them. Yet the links between our addiction to industrial milk and meat consumption and escalating cancer rates can no longer be ignored. Not surprisingly, the American Public Health Association voted to support a ban on US hormonal milk and hormonal meat in 2009. And, not surprisingly, our milk and meat are banned in the European Union, in addition to many other nations worldwide. What does this tell us about the safety of the food that we consume, and feed our children, morning, noon, and night?

How did we get here? In recent years, the food health dialogue in Washington has continued to be influenced and controlled the agricultural and food industrial complex headed by such megacorporations as Monsanto, Carville, and Hormel. We cannot wait for federal health officials to assure us that we are consuming healthy and safe foods; rather, we must protect ourselves by being informed consumers. This book serves up a wakeup call, a warning that eating a standard American diet, rich in hormonal meat and dairy, poses a threat to your health. Just as importnatly, it offers practical steps to take to minimize your risk and stay safe. With decades of medical research behind him, as well as numerous interactions with America's health establishment and the country's leading medical associations, Dr. Epstein intimately knows what families are up against and why average foods are endangering the lives of the nation's children and adults. It is time for families to better educate themselves about the foods they purchase, what they order in restaurants and put on their plates. This book is an important contribution in guiding us in the right direction.

The good news is that science supporting the benefits of wholesome products and the health risks of commercial meat, dairy, and genetically modified crops and vegetables are increasing dramatically. More and more physicians, health experts, and nutritionists—even the media—are coming around to appreciating the medical benefits of good clean food and the dangers of industrialized food products. Certified organic meat and milk are becoming more widely available and more affordable, and recent national polls show Americans are gradually beginning to avoid industrial milk and meat altogether.

As we sit back and witness food allergies, asthma, diabetes, weakened immune systems, and a host of other disorders and illnesses reach epidemic proportions in American children, *Good Clean Food* should be required reading for every parent and school teacher. The book should also be required reading for every federal and state legislator and health official. There is still time to save our younger generations from the consequences of the previous generations' errors, a blind faith in Big Agro-Chemical industry's false promises. I believe Dr. Epstein has written a book that contributes to the reform necessary to turn the tide on our declining national health and to restore the health, vitality, peace of mind, and well-being to all families and their children. But its immediate effects lie with you, the consumer, and the informed choices you will make the next time you stand at the end of the supermarket aisle, wondering what's for dinner.

CHAPTER 1
An Introduction

When we stroll down the supermarket aisles, we are faced with a myriad of products: organic, all-natural, pesticide-free, grass-fed, rBGH-free, non-GMO, artificial hormone-free, and so on. We spend a lot of time staring at the cartons and the cans and the plastic packaging, trying to pick the nutritious foods that will fuel a long and productive life for ourselves and for our children, without putting undue strain on our wallets.

But GMOs—genetically modified organisms—threaten that picture.

More than 60 percent of the items on supermarket shelves, almost one item in three, contains genetically modified ingredients. We're discussing just about everything from infant formula to corn chips, notes John Hagelin, PhD, Director of the Institute of Science, Technology and Public Policy and International Director of the Global Union of Scientists for Peace. Moreover, Hagelin points out, none of these foods have been safety tested on humans, and none are labeled. (Labeling is, of course, a separate issue, which we discuss in chapter 9: "Future Trends," page 123.)

By now, most Americans are well aware of the controversy regarding GMOs in general and recombinant Bovine Growth Hormone (rBGH) in particular. We know how scientific laboratories can modify a whole range of organisms, from microorganisms such as bacteria and yeast, to larger organisms such as plants, fish, and even mammals. We've seen studies that trace increased rates of cancer to our food system, and we've also read about researchers who find the studies unconvincing and the results inconclusive. And we've wondered about what all this has to do with our milk, our meat, our fruits and vegetables.

There is, in fact, so much information out there about genetically modified organisms that it can be overwhelming. Think about it: if people with a doctorate in microbiology haven't been able to clearly decide one way or the other, have trouble weighing this scientific study against that one and against a third, how can people with a little bit of high school or college biology sort out the details and make the right decisions?

What we put in our bodies is not just a once-in-a-while decision, relegated to when we have the time and energy to devote to research and thought. We "vote" with our stomachs on this very personal environmental issue every time we sit down for breakfast, lunch, and dinner, not to mention when we decide, perhaps against our better judgment, to have a snack. We vote every time we respond to the perennial, "Mom, I'm hungry." But with all the information—and misinformation—out there, it is hard to vote knowledgeably. This book will clarify some of these issues so you can choose foods that will actually nourish your body as well as fill your stomach.

Why It Matters

The US Environmental Protection Agency (EPA) has registered nearly fourteen hundred pesticides for agricultural and nonagricultural use. These chemicals include approximately forty that have been classified by the International Agency for Research on Cancer (IARC) as known, probable, or possible carcinogens, according to the *2008–09 Annual Report President's Cancer Panel: Reducing Environmental Cancer Risk: What We Can Do Now.*

Exposure to these chemicals has been linked to a range of cancers, including brain and central nervous system (CNS), colon, lung, breast and ovarian (female spouses), pancreatic, kidney, testicular, and stomach cancers, as well as Hodgkin's and non-Hodgkin's lymphoma, multiple myeloma, and soft tissue sarcoma, notes the report. In addition, people who are involved more directly with these pesticides—such as crop duster pilots, manufacturers, and farmers who apply the products—have been found to have greater risk of prostate cancer, melanoma, and other skin cancers, as well as cancer of the lip.

Clearly, these pesticides carry at least a hint of danger. Pesticides were designed in the first place to kill pests; how, then, can they be good for human beings? The question, rather, is whether there is any residue of these chemicals left in the food by the time it shows up on our dining room tables.

To determine the level of pesticide residue left in our food, the US Department of Agriculture (USDA) samples more than eighty types of fruits, vegetables, nuts, meats, grains, dairy products, and other foods regularly to see whether—and how much—pesticide, herbicide, fungicide, and growth regulators the foods contain. In the most recent report, the Department of Agriculture found that 18.5 percent of the foods sampled contained one pesticide, and 40.5 percent contained more than one pesticide.[1] The foods we eat, the foods we serve, are not as pure and chemical-free as we'd like.

Top Pesticide: Atrazine

In the United States, atrazine holds the dubious honor of being the leading pesticide contaminant of groundwater, surface water, and drinking water, according to the President's Cancer Panel. Produced by Syngenta AG, a Swiss-based chemical company, atrazine is designed to kill broadleaf and grassy weeds and has been banned for use by the European Union. Despite the fact that its own country, its own continent, has found it dangerous, the United States continues to import the chemical and use it to produce our food.

The US Environmental Protection Agency (EPA) has analyzed atrazine, which is used mostly in the Midwest on corn, sorghum, and sugarcane, and has concluded that while there are "areas of concern"—including cancer—simply regulating the US drinking water should protect Americans adequately from any harmful residues of the chemical. By contrast, the National Cancer Institute (NCI) has also looked at the pesticide and determines that "both animal and human studies have suggested that atrazine is possibly carcinogenic," and recommends further study. There is not yet enough data to decide one way or the other, states the NCI.

This is a classic case of conscientious scientists unable to come to an agreement, leaving consumers in the dark. So, while the EPA and the NCI can agree to disagree, in light of the EU ban, the questions for consumers remain: What do we want in our food? What is an "acceptable level of risk" to put into our bodies on a daily basis? And what do we want to feed to our children?

How Did We Get Here?

It was only about a hundred years ago that almost half of all Americans (about 40 percent) lived on farms. Most food was bought and eaten locally, according to the season, and people generally knew where their food came from, according to the USDA. Chances are, even people who didn't live on farms bumped into the farmers at school PTA meetings or in the local post office.

After World War II, America shifted from this local food system to more of a national, and then even international, system. Highways improved, refrigerated trucking got cheaper, other forms of transportation became more feasible, and soon even perishables such as meat, eggs, fruits, and vegetables could be easily shipped across state and country lines and around the globe. Different areas began to specialize in growing particular foods, notes the USDA; for instance, fruits and tree nuts became concentrated in California and Florida. We had separated people from the food they eat. By the year 2000, only about 1 percent of Americans lived on farms. Children are growing up thinking that chickens have fingers.

Not only were the relationships between farms and consumers changing, but the farms themselves transformed, becoming increasingly efficient and productive. New technology—such as motors and pumps, electric milking parlors, and grain elevators—enhanced efficiency. Advances in fertilizers and herbicides reduced waste, and new approaches to plant and animal breeding boosted production. The American agricultural landscape changed, with fewer—and much larger—farms taking the place of what used to be ubiquitous family businesses. Along the way came genetically modified organisms (GMOs), which have played a vital role in this process.

Genetically modified organisms were designed by chemical companies here and abroad to meet an important need. With today's world population at about seven billion, there is increasing concern about how to feed all those people. In fact, the Organization for Economic Cooperation and Development (OECD), based in Paris, states that agricultural production will need to increase by 60 percent over the next forty years in order to meet the rising demand for food. Some experts worry that traditional food production just can't provide enough nutrition for this burgeoning population.

In steps the notion of genetic modification.

The GMO Story

Genetic modification is actually nothing new. When Gregor Mendel figured out the role of genes in passing along traits, in the late 1800s, he gave us some more tools, paving the way for the first genetically modified plant. Since then, people have been crossbreeding related plant or animal species to improve taste or productivity. The Mendelian approach, though, is very time-consuming because it can take several generations to gain—or lose—a particular trait.

Things really got cracking in the crop modification arena when James D. Watson and Francis Crick discovered the structure of DNA, describing the double helix and the notion of DNA-encoded genes in 1954. The science of molecular biology was born. Researchers kept plugging away for another two decades until, in 1973, Stanley Cohen at Stanford and Herbert Boyer at the University of California, San Francisco created the first recombinant DNA molecules by cutting up a DNA sequence and putting it back together again.

These days, genetic modification typically takes place in a chemical company laboratory. Tissue samples from the organism to be modified are placed in a culture, and one or more genetically modified genes are placed into that tissue. The goal is to reprogram the genetic blueprint of the original tissue, giving it completely new properties—often a resistance to herbicides or pesticides. Not all of the cells in the tissue sample pick up the new genes, so the next step is to get rid of those that lack the new qualities and help the remaining tissue grow into a full-fledged, genetically modified plant.

This is an artificial process, according to Earth Open Source, a nonprofit organization dedicated to assuring the sustainability, security, and safety of the global food system. But, notes the organization, it is not necessarily an inherently dangerous one; the results are often crude and unpredictable. They are also irreversible; unlike with a chemical cloud that will eventually dissipate, a genetically modified organism will continue to reproduce itself.

Monsanto, arguably the leading biotechnology company in the world, claims that genetically breeding traits into organisms—such as adding herbicide or insecticide tolerance—can boost crop yields by protecting the crops from losses due to insects or weeds. According to Monsanto, herbicide-tolerant soybeans have increased yields in Romania by 31 percent; virus-resistant papaya has increased yields by an average of 40 percent in Hawaii; and insect-resistant cotton has led to yield increases of more than 50 percent in India.

Proponents of GMOs suggest that there are several additional reasons to turn to these food sources: in addition to increasing the amount of food produced, they provide more environmentally friendly food production, and more nutritious foods. And proponents say that GMOs are perfectly safe, within governmentally regulated limits.

Do GMOs Really Increase Crop Production?

The Union of Concerned Scientists, a nonprofit organization that combines rigorous, independent science with advocacy work, refutes the assertion that GMOs increase food production. The organization says that the only GMO food or feed crops that have shown significantly improved yield are varieties of Bt corn—and that the increases they have seen are less than what we've gained from conventionally grown corn. And, as we will see later, GMO crops don't do very well in drought conditions, such as those that often exist in the parts of the world most in desperate need of increased food.

We shouldn't pin our hopes on GMOs to solve the crisis of world hunger.

The Bigger Question

Beyond that, though, there remains the bigger question: Do we want to put these chemicals into our bodies?

GMOs are part of many, many foods sold in this country. Americans, in 2012, ate their weight or more in genetically engineered foods, and do so each year, according to an Environmental Working Group analysis of US government data. The group found that Americans eat an average of 193 pounds of genetically engineered food over a twelve-month period. That's more than the typical US adult weight of 179 pounds. When we're eating that much of something, it's probably a good idea to know what it is.

Others argue that we do not know enough about the safety of these foods, that they are typically not labeled as GMO, so we are buying blind, and that there is insufficient oversight and control of their production and distribution. They argue that the GMO movement is fueled not by an altruistic attempt to feed the world, but by corporate greed designed to boost the income of multinational corporations. *Good Clean Food* will provide the information you need to make those vital decisions for yourself and your family.

The Organic Food Movement

The organic food movement in the United States began with a handful of well-intentioned farmers looking to farm in a way that would be better for the land and healthier for themselves and for the people eating the food. Organic farmers tried to encourage soil and water conservation and used alternative methods for fertilizing, controlling weeds, and preventing live-stock disease. For instance, notes the Mayo Clinic, organic farmers may use crop rotations and mulch instead of weed killers to keep weeds out of the fields. Different organic farmers use different methods, depending on their climate and crops and even personal preference.

At the beginning of the organic food movement, organic food was sold only in natural food stores, in small quantities, and usually carrying high price tags. Organic aficionados tended to live "alternative lifestyles," and they often had a relationship with the farmers and retailers that provided their food. These people shopped organic for a variety of reasons. Some simply preferred the taste of organic food. Others were more focused on avoiding pesticides, food additives, and other items of concern, such as antibiotics. Antibiotics are a particular concern, according to *Environmental Health*, because about 70 percent of the antibiotics used in the United States each year are used as feed additives for chickens, hogs, and beef cattle—not to treat disease, but to promote growth.

Still other people interested in organic food were worried about the effect of pesticides and antibiotic use, not just on themselves and their families, but on the larger environment. At this point, both organic farmers and organic consumers were a small but committed group.

Organic Goes Mainstream

Over time, organic has gone mainstream. According to the Center for Sustainable and Agricultural Resources at Washington State University, the US organic food industry has been growing between 20 percent and 30 percent a year over the past decade; in the state of Washington, for instance, organic acreage has increased eight-fold since 1993.

The growth of organic food is not just concentrated in Washington State, though. More and more farmers are using organic farming techniques; greater numbers of supermarkets, groceries, and even restaurants are selling organic food; and more and more Americans are filling their refrigerators with organic items. (See the appendix, starting on page 145 for lists of rBGH-free dairy product suppliers, organic soy producers, organic egg producers, and hormone-free and grass-fed beef suppliers around the country.) The challenge for the consumer, though, is that different producers use different labels to describe their products, which makes it difficult to comparison shop, or sometimes even to figure out precisely what is contained in each "organic" food item.

We have seen that organic food offers benefits beyond the mere absence of pesticides and antibiotics. For instance, a 2012 study by Alyson Mitchell, PhD, and colleagues published in the *Journal of Agricultural and Food Chemistry*, found that organic spinach has lower levels of nitrates and higher levels of flavanoids and ascorbic acid, both known for their antioxidant qualities.[2] Another group of researchers found that organic tomatoes and peppers have more vitamin C than their nonorganic peers.[3] Yet another study found that organic peaches, pears, strawberries, marionberries, and sweet corn have higher levels of flavonoids and ascorbic acid than their conventionally grown counterparts.[4] These differences are apparent even after accounting for the varying agricultural practices among both organic and traditional growing techniques.

Federal Regulation

Toward the end of the twentieth century, the federal government stepped in to regulate the "organic" products on American supermarket shelves. In 1990, Congress passed the Organic Foods Production Act (the Act), as part of the 1990 Farm Bill. This bill is considered one of the strongest of the US public health laws, according to the Environmental Working Group. It emphasizes protecting infants, children, and other vulnerable people.

This bill recruited the USDA for the job. The USDA was to establish national standards for the production and handling of organic products to assure consumers that agricultural products marketed as "organic" meet consistent, uniform standards. It also set up an organic certification program and a National Organic Standards Board, appointed by the Secretary of Agriculture. The National Organic Program was charged with developing, implementing, and administering national standards on the marketing and production of agricultural products; it keeps track of what is allowed—and what is not allowed—in producing and handling organic foods. The regulations were finalized in December 2000, just in time for the new millennium.

Setting the Standard

The National Organic Standard became law on October 21, 2002. It sets out a national standard for the term "organic." Organic food must be produced without conventional pesticides, petroleum-based fertilizers, sewage sludge-based fertilizers, herbicides, pesticides, genetic engineering (biotechnology), antibiotics, growth hormones, or irradiation. Animals raised on an organic farm must be fed organic feed and given access to the outdoors. And the land itself must be "organic"; it must have had no prohibited substances applied to it for at least three years before the harvest of an officially "organic" crop. To display the USDA Organic seal, farms and handling operations must be certified by a state or private agency. While the USDA imprimatur is not perfect, it is, at least, consistent state to state and product to product and assures customers of a minimum standard of "organic."

There are also a few variations on the theme. Here are the terms:

- *100 percent Organic* means all ingredients and processing aids are organic.
- *Organic* means all agricultural products must be certified as organic and there can be specified nonorganic ingredients (those on the national list) that may represent up to a total of 5 percent of the content.

- *Made with Organic Ingredients* means that at least 70 percent of the product must be certified organic ingredients and any nonorganic ingredients must be specifically allowed on the national list.

Products that aren't labeled as USDA-certified Organic can still contain organic ingredients, but chances are, they'll have less than 70 percent certified-organic ingredients.

Psychology of Greed

The image of the multinational corporation looms large in the American psyche, and many people worry that these corporations place their profit goals ahead of human life. Newspaper headlines regularly support this notion, with constant references to pollution, child labor, unfair wages, and unsafe methods of production. Whatever the goal of the multinational corporations involved in production of genetically modified organisms, though, it is hard to deny that the trend has resulted in major corporate profits. It is equally difficult to refute the observation that there is at least a serious question of ill effects on the people who eat these foods.

Many people have a hard time understanding how companies can knowingly make choices that might endanger the lives of fellow Americans. Why would a company, for instance, place an additional dollar's worth of profit over the health of our children? Surely, for instance, maintaining sanitary animal pens is easier, cheaper, and safer than irradiating the meat after the fact.

Some psychologists suggest that there is some uniquely American quality that encourages this behavior. They propose that America's emphasis on materialism promotes behavior that could—and, in some cases, does—lead to taking health risks with our national health. "Our form of capitalism encourages materialistic values, and the research shows that people high on materialism . . . are more likely to engage in unethical business behaviors and manipulate people for their own purposes," social psychologist Tim Kasser, PhD, of Knox College in Galesburg, Illinois, was quoted as saying in an article in the magazine *Psychology Today*.

Cross-cultural studies make the indictment even stronger. American culture is different than that of other English-speaking countries, notes psychologist Shalom Schwartz, PhD, at Hebrew University of Jerusalem, because it emphasizes mastery and hierarchy more than intellectual autonomy, harmony, and egalitarianism. This orientation, he notes, encourages an assertive, pragmatic, entrepreneurial, and even exploitative approach toward the social and natural environment. The Horatio Alger motif, the notion of "making it in America," in other words, can sometimes beat out the idea that "we're all in this together."

Organic Is Growing

Fortunately, not everyone is affected by this mindset. Many people *do* believe that we are all in this together. Indeed, organic farms are a growing force in American agriculture, according to the USDA. As of 2011, there were a total of 9,140 USDA-certified organic farms in the United States, representing a total of 3.6 million organic acres. The top four organic-farm states are California (with 1,898 farms), Wisconsin (870), New York (597), Washington (493), and Iowa (with 467 farms). The US organic-farm sector consists of a broad mix of farm sizes and production specialties and includes many farms that manage both conventional and organic crops and livestock operations.

There is no typical organic farmer, though, observes the USDA. If anything, data from the survey show that certified and exempt organic farmers, on average, tend to operate smaller farms (280 acres) than other US farmers (418 acres). Organic agriculture also has a higher share of female farm and ranch operators (22 percent, compared with 14 percent for conventional agriculture) and younger operators (the average age was fifty-three for organic farms and fifty-seven for all farmers overall).

And So Are the Customers

More and more Americans are buying organic food. For starters, it's much easier to do it these days than it used to be. Once available only in natural product stores and farmers' markets, organic foods can now be found in conventional supermarkets, value-priced, big-box chains, and an expanding array of direct-to-consumer markets, such as community supported agriculture. (See chapter 9.) Without going out of the way or making an extra stop in our hectic lives, most Americans can now choose between traditionally grown apples, for instance, and organic ones, as we fill up our shopping carts.

Availability makes it easier but, really, the top reasons that Americans cite for going organic are that they prefer to eat food without pesticides (cited by 64 percent); herbicides (60 percent); growth hormones (59 percent); artificial flavors, colors, and preservatives (56 percent); antibiotics (55 percent); genetically modified organisms (54 percent); and irradiation (48 percent), according to the Seattle-based Hartman Group, a market research firm. In short, the benefits of organic food are important—but even more critical is the absence of harmful materials that are typically present in conventional foods.

The numbers help tell the story. Total sales of organic food in 2011 totaled $3.53 billion, including crops ($2.2 billion, or 62.9 percent of the total) and livestock and poultry ($1.31 billion). The average sales per farm, according to the USDA, was $414,726 in 2011, a huge increase from the 2007 figure of $134,807 per farm.

Of course, not every state is as heavily invested in organic food. People who live on the West Coast seem to be more interested in going organic than the rest of the country, according to the Hartman Group. The top state for sale of certified organic food in 2011, far and away, was California, responsible for 39.3 percent of the total. The next biggest organic buyers were Washington State (8.4 percent), Oregon (6.6 percent), Texas (4.7 percent), and Wisconsin (3.8 percent).

Even within localities, people vary in their commitment to eating organic, according to the *SPINSscan Consumer* report, produced by SPINS, a consulting firm focused on the organic market. The report found, not surprisingly, that people most committed to organic food are buying more organic, and those people who only buy organic occasionally are doing so less often. More specifically, SPINS found, over the year 2008 to

2009, the 20 percent of consumers most committed to buying organic spent 12.6 percent more on organic food than before; the middle quarter of consumers spent an additional 12 percent; and the remaining 55 percent actually cut their organic expenses—but only by 1.6 percent.

A Preview of the Book

Good Clean Food offers up-to-date information that you need to make the best food choices for you and your family. It goes through food group by food group, topic by topic, and presents the scientific data you need to help you make these decisions.

Two of the most contentious battlegrounds are the dairy industry (chapter 2: "Got Milk," page 17) and the meat industry (chapter 3: "Where's the Beef?" page 35). This book devotes a chapter to each of those subjects, outlining some of the most relevant scientific studies. Chapter 4 ("The Dirty Dozen," page 53) looks specifically at fruits and vegetables, asking the question: If you can't afford to buy all organic, what are the most important food items to focus on? And, conversely, what conventionally grown items are most likely to be safe? Then we take a chapter to look at the role of GMOs in grains, specifically corn and soybean in "Going Against the Grain" (chapter 5, page 71). Chapter 6: "Which Came First, the Chicken or the Egg?" (page 87) looks at the issues associated with organic and free-range eggs. Each of these chapters tells the reader what the potential concerns are, what the research shows, and how to feed your family safely.

There's a lot of information in the food-specific chapters. But how do you incorporate all those scientific studies and research surveys into your daily life? The last several chapters focus on figuring out how to make use of all of this information.

Chapter 7 ("Avoiding GMOs," page 97) provides a series of practical steps that we can take to avoid consuming GMOs and other unwanted chemicals. Chapter 8 ("Detoxification: Nutritional and Dietary Approaches," page 107) addresses actions that we can take to adapt our lifestyles to better meet our nutritional needs and to detoxify and heal our bodies, including a series of complementary and alternative medical (CAM) therapies. Finally, chapter 9 looks to the future of GMOs and healthy eating. It considers shopping organic on a budget; the changing demographics of organic aficionados; the contentious topic of mandatory labeling; taking the challenge of avoiding GMOs a step further; and the worldwide response to the issue of genetically modified organisms.

As more and more supermarkets, grocery stores, restaurants, and other food retailers provide organic options to consumers, access becomes easier and sales rise. And as sales of organic foods rise, the cost of producing these safer, healthier food options goes down. American consumers are not giving in to the drive toward corporate greed. We are learning to—we must—vote with our stomachs and make informed decisions about the food that we eat, the food we serve to our children.

CHAPTER 2

Got Milk?

The US Dietary Guidelines recommend that children between the ages of one and eight have at least two servings a day of milk and other dairy products; starting at age nine and up through adulthood, the guidelines recommend three servings a day. A serving of dairy can be an eight-ounce glass of milk, but it can also be eight ounces of yogurt or soymilk, one and a half ounces of natural cheese, or two ounces of processed cheese. (Bear in mind that there is controversy over whether dairy is actually required or whether the human body simply needs sufficient calcium, defined by the National Institutes of Health as 1,000 mg a day for adults. Calcium is also plentiful in a range of nondairy products, such as broccoli, sardines, and salmon.) In general, Americans seem to have no trouble consuming enough calcium. According to *Advertising Age Magazine*, the average American knocks back 20.4 gallons of milk a year, which should have us covered, calcium-wise. But is that all we're consuming, as we sip the white, creamy beverage?

The BGH Story

As we saw in chapter 1, the concept of genetically modified organisms is nothing new in human history. Ever since humans settled down into agrarian societies, we have been domesticating crops and animals to suit our needs, increase production, and make food taste better.

When it comes specifically to the milk industry, dairy farmers have long had a trick up their sleeves. Bovine growth hormone (BGH) is a naturally occurring protein hormone produced in the cow's pituitary glands that promotes growth and cell replication. (Incidentally, BGH is also produced in other animals, including human beings.) As early as 1937, dairy farmers knew that naturally occurring bovine somatotropin (abbreviated bST and BST), also known as BGH, could increase milk yield in lactating cows by preventing mammary cell death in dairy cattle.

But there was only so much naturally occurring BGH to go around; the only source, for years, was bovine cadavers, an unreliable and slightly icky way to boost milk yield. The industry needed another, more reliable source of this hormone to fully take advantage of BGH's production-enhancing qualities.

In the Beginning, Genentech Created . . .

In the 1970s, Genentech, a biotechnology company, developed a genetically engineered "recombinant" version of the protein hormone. In a science laboratory, researchers cloned the rBGH gene into the bacteria *E. coli*, grew that artificially created bacteria, and then separated out and purified the rBGH. Genentech worked together with Monsanto, another multinational chemical company, to figure out the best way to use this artificial hormone on a farm. Together, the two companies determined that injecting this hormone into a lactating cow would boost milk production by somewhere between 10 percent and 15 percent.

Now that the milk-enhancing protein could be produced synthetically, there were new possibilities for boosting bovine milk production. All that was necessary was a manufacturer, and, of course, regulatory approval from the appropriate authorities. The corporate world—specifically Monsanto, American Cyanamid, Eli Lilly, and Upjohn—raced to develop commercial rBGH products and submit them to the FDA for approval. Lilly won the race to market, with sales in Mexico and Brazil. Monsanto licensed Genentech's patent, then named their product Posilac.

Enter Posilac

The FDA assessed Posilac, reviewing the safety and efficacy data. The Vermont Public Interest Group and Rural Vermont questioned the data, according to the FDA. But the FDA determined that food products from cows treated with rBGH are perfectly safe for us to eat. On November 5, 1993, the FDA approved rBGH for use in the agricultural industry. In 1994, Monsanto brought Posilac to the market. In October 2008, Monsanto sold this business, in full, to Lilly for a cool $300 million plus "additional considerations."

People were less excited about rBGH on the other side of the Atlantic Ocean. Michael H. Erhard of the Ludwig-Maximilians-Universität München in Bavaria, Germany, reported evidence that rBGH is immunologically different from natural BGH in the *Journal of Immunoassay*. In April 1990, the European Union (EU) declared a provisional ban on the use and marketing of rBGH and debated the issue at an International Milk Day Convention in Bonn, Germany. Two years later, after much consideration, the European Council reaffirmed its moratorium on rBGH, which meant the discussion was not yet final—but it was getting close.

Similarly, Canada was also concerned about rBGH. At the request of Health Canada, the Canadian Veterinary Medical Association (CVMA) and the Royal College of Physicians and Surgeons established an Expert Panel to review the efficacy and safety of rBGH. The panel confirmed that rBGH does, in fact, increase milk yield by an average of 11.3 percent in cows pregnant for the first time, and even more, approximately 15.6 percent, in cows that have already given birth two or more times. So in terms of efficacy, rBGH performed exactly as billed.

But the Canadian researchers found that rBGH also increased the risk of clinical mastitis by approximately 25 percent, caused a variety of reproductive concerns (cystic ovaries, twinning, retained placenta, and fetal loss), and led to a 50 percent increase in the risk of clinical lameness. Not reassuring. Ultimately, on January 14, 1999, Health Canada banned all use of rBGH within its borders.

Some American firms agreed with European and Canadian concerns about rBGH. In 1993, Ben and Jerry's Ice Cream announced that it would label its ice cream explicitly to assure consumers that the milk and cream used came from cooperatives or farmers who had not used rBGH. For a while, the company displayed illustrations of dairy cows with signs hung around their necks that declared "rBGH free, that's me!" The next issue within the US borders was labeling: Would milk produced using the artificial hormone rBGH be labeled as such? Or would the packaging look just like milk produced the old-fashioned way? In 1994, the FDA approved the sale of unlabeled rBGH milk in the United States. As soon as sale within its own borders was legal, the United States encouraged Mexico and other trading partners to approve rBGH in their countries, focusing on the World Trade Organization. (In general, the United States isn't fond of labeling genetically modified organisms; see chapter 9: "Future Trends," page 123.)

International Concerns

The United States is not the only place that has deemed GMOs to be safe for human consumption. The Food and Agriculture/World Health Organization's (FAO/WHO) Joint Expert Committees on Food Additives (JECFA) agrees. JECFA produced a report on rBGH in 1998, reporting the hormone as safe, which was approved by the Codex Committee on Residues of Veterinary Drugs in Foods. It is noteworthy that at this point, the chair of JECFA was FDA's Director for Veterinary Medicine, Stephen Sundloff, DVM, PhD.

Then the United Nations entered into the fray. On August 18, 1999, the *Codex Alimentarius* Commission, the UN Food Safety Agency representing 101 nations, ruled unanimously in favor of the 1993 European moratorium on Monsanto's genetically engineered hormonal milk (rBGH). As a result, the United States opted not to challenge the European moratorium before the World Trade Organization. The UN decision represents the first time genetically modified foods were rejected for scientific grounds, rather than for ethical or ideological concerns.

Meanwhile, the European Commission wanted to take a good look at the situation, to make a final decision about its moratorium. It commissioned two independent committees of internationally recognized experts to undertake a comprehensive review of the scientific literature on both the veterinary and public health effects of rBGH. The first committee, focusing on veterinary issues, fully confirmed and extended the Canadian warnings and conclusions. The second committee, looking at public health concerns, confirmed earlier reports of higher-than-expected levels of the naturally occurring Insulin-like-Growth Factor One (IGF-1), including its potent variants, in rBGH milk; this committee concluded that IGF-1 posed major risks of cancer, particularly of the breast and prostate, promoting the growth and invasiveness of cancer cells by inhibiting their programmed, self-destruction (apoptosis). On January 1, 2000, the EU converted its 1990 moratorium on the use and marketing of rBGH into a formal ban. Case closed for the European Union.

Given the research and decisions in both Canada and Europe, the United States opted not to question the *Codex Alimentarius* Commission decision. But that didn't mean there was going to be a change within the US borders.

Here, the controversy continued. On June 8, 2000, the FDA denied the Center for Food Safety's citizens petition to remove rBGH from the American market. Then, on December 18, a blue ribbon, joint US-EU Biotechnology Consulting Forum urged that "at the very least, consumers should have the right of informed choice." More specifically, the Forum recommended the establishment of "content-based mandatory requirements for finished products containing novel genetic material."

In November 2009, the Governing Council of the American Public Health Association voted to oppose the continued sale and use of rBGH milk. Despite this statement, rBGH was, and remains, in use coast to coast in this country.

Looking at Posilac

Monsanto's version of injectable rBGH is—as we've said—named Posilac. At this point, it is estimated that approximately 20 percent of all American dairy farmers inject their cows regularly with rBGH in the form of Posilac.

In the package insert, the FDA lays out a very specific process for administering Posilac to cows. Dairy farmers inject one syringe of Posilac every fourteen days beginning the ninth or tenth week (between fifty-seven and seventy days) after calving and continue until the end of lactation. Recommended injection sites are in the neck area behind the shoulder or in the depression on either side of the tail head. The FDA instructions include the following warning to farmers:

> Avoid prolonged or repeated contact of Posilac with eyes and skin. Posilac is a protein. Frequent skin contact with proteins in general may produce an allergic skin reaction in some people. Always wash hands and skin exposed to Posilac with soap and water after handling. Clothing soiled with the product should be laundered before reuse.

According to the FDA, Posilac can cause a number of side effects for the cows receiving the hormone, as well. Swelling of up to four inches in diameter can occur at the injection site, and this condition may well remain permanent. Posilac can also lead to overall health problems, such as increased body temperature and heat stress, as well as increased incidence of clinical or subclinical mastitis. The hormone can also affect cows' reproductive abilities. It can, for instance, lower pregnancy rates, increase incidence of retained placenta, decrease gestation length, lower birth rate, boost rate of twin births, and can also lead to cystic ovaries or other disorders of the uterus.

Some side effects are unrelated to reproduction. Posilac can cause cows to have digestive disorders, including indigestion, bloating, diarrhea, and decreased appetite. It can also cause enlarged hocks and knee lesions and disorders of the feet. Internally, it can affect the cow's blood, leading to reduced levels of hemoglobin or hematocrit. And some of these side effects—as well as the substances used to treat them—get passed on to the people who drink the milk.

Pus in the Milk

Since cows receiving Posilac are much more likely to contract mastitis—25 percent more likely, according to Health Canada—rBGH milk often contains more pus than hormone-free milk. And, of course, the mastitis must be treated. So, in addition to pus, the milk may well contain residue of the antibiotics and possibly other veterinary drugs used to treat the mastitis. Some farmers even treat mastitis prophylactically—in advance of any observable problem—with low-level antibiotics. That approach means that consumers may be drinking even more antibiotics than are absolutely necessary, even with the use of Posilac. Some scientists are concerned that all of these antibiotics in the milk could play into the rise of antibiotic-resistant bacteria in this country and possibly worldwide.

How much of these antibiotics are we talking about? It's hard to get a precise figure. The Public Broadcasting System (PBS), in its *Frontline* series, maintains that farmers have been feeding small doses of antibiotics to cows for years because they discovered that such a "subtherapeutic" dose will cause the animals to gain as much as 3 percent more weight than they would otherwise. And that's before we even throw rBGH into the equation.

In 2002, a study published in the *Journal of Antimicrobial Chemotherapy* by Stuart B. Levy, MD, Director of the Center for Adaptation Genetics and Drug Resistance at Tufts University School of Medicine, found that we use about seven billion kg of antibiotics, chiefly penicillins and tetracyclines, to promote growth in farm animals.

Researchers Andrew Charles Zwald, Pamela L. Ruegg, and several of their colleagues at the University of Wisconsin–Madison found in a

2004 study that the vast majority of dairy farmers (84.9 percent) gave up to 10 percent of their cows antibiotics, and 9.1 percent gave antibiotics to as much as a quarter of the herd. And that is for healthy cattle. In contrast, almost all organic farmers (90.6 percent) reported no antibiotic use at all. The researchers also found that 79.8 percent of dairy farmers gave antibiotics to cows to treat mastitis; in the course of this study, organic farmers did not give a single treatment of antibiotics for mastitis to their herds.[5] In other words, there's a good chance that your kids are drinking antibiotics along with their after-school snack of milk and cookies.

And this extensive use of antibiotics can also lead to antibiotic resistance. Antibiotics have been enormously useful in treating a wide range of illnesses—human illnesses—over the years. But they've been around so long that the infectious organisms—the "bugs" that antibiotics have been designed to treat—have adapted to the antibiotics. They've built up a resistance, making the drugs less effective, notes the CDC. People who are infected with antibiotic-resistant organisms often end up in a hospital for a long stay—and they may be more likely to die from the infection, adds the CDC.

Bacteria can also develop cross-resistance, which occurs when their resistance to one drug also makes them resistant to other, related drugs. This does happen, according to the Union of Concerned Scientists, and occurred in Europe with vancomycin. That was a drug that had been used as a last resort for treating certain life-threatening infections. To try to avoid the development of antibiotic-resistant bugs, the scientific community recommends more careful and judicious use of antibiotics. Giving prophylactic antibiotics to livestock may not be the best way to achieve that goal.

Reproductive Concerns

Drinking rBGH milk can affect a woman's reproductive system as well as a cow's reproductive system. A June 27, 2006, study by Dr. Gary Steinman published in the *Journal of Reproductive Medicine* reported that women drinking milk and eating dairy products from cows injected with the hormone are up to five times more likely to risk giving birth to fraternal twins than women who don't consume dairy products. The study also showed that rBGH milk is not the same as milk from cows who have not been injected with rBGH. The rBGH milk contains several abnormalities, including reduced levels of casein and short-chain fatty acids, as well as increased levels of long-chain fatty acid levels and thyroid hormone triiodothyronine enzyme.

Insulin-Like Growth Factor 1

Posilac causes elevated concentrations of insulin-like growth factor 1 (IGF-1) in cows and their milk, up to 8 ug per liter of milk. In fact, it can contain up to ten times more than in natural milk. IGF-1 is readily absorbed through the small intestine and poses increased risks of breast, colon, and childhood cancers.

Now, we know that milk isn't always perfect; that's why we pasteurize it. Pasteurization involves heating milk to below-boiling temperature in order to kill harmful organisms that are responsible for such diseases as listeriosis, typhoid fever, tuberculosis, diphtheria, and brucellosis, according to the FDA.

Unfortunately, IGF-1 is not destroyed by pasteurization. In fact, pasteurization actually increases the IGF-1 levels in milk. Digestion doesn't destroy the hormone, either. Rather, IGF-1 is readily absorbed across the intestinal wall and can move its way into the bloodstream, where it can affect other hormones.

The problem with IGF-1's presence in standard milk is, basically, that IGF-1 encourages cells to grow. A Harvard Medical School study shows that when IGF-1 is added to dishes of cells growing in the laboratory, the cells flourish. In children, IGF-1 stimulates bone growth and the development of organs such as the heart, liver, and kidneys.

In adults, though, rapidly growing cells isn't always a good thing. In fact, pretty much past childhood, rapidly proliferating cells tend to increase the opportunity for genetic mutations that can lead to cancer.

Once cancer cells begin to form, IGF-1 will encourage them to grow, alongside normal cells.[6]

A May 9, 1998, article in the *Lancet* reported that women with a relatively small increase in blood levels of IGF-1 are up to seven times more likely to develop premenopausal breast cancer than women with lower levels. The report concluded that the risks of elevated IGF-1 blood levels are among the leading known risk factors for breast cancer; the only bigger risks are a strong family history or an unusual mammogram result. The 1998 Harvard Nurses' Health Study, for instance, showed that those with elevated IGF-1 blood levels experienced up to a seven-fold increased risk of breast cancer.

More recent studies have had similar findings. A 2010 study in the *Lancet* found that circulating IGF-1 is positively associated with breast cancer risk, according to author Timothy J. Key at the Nuffield Department of Clinical Medicine, University of Oxford, and colleagues. The study also found that IGF-1 is mostly associated with estrogen-receptor-positive tumors (which represent approximately 75 percent of all breast cancers).[7]

And it's not just breast cancer. A study of more than three thousand people from eight European countries found that high circulating IGF-1 concentration is positively associated with risk for prostate cancer over the short and long term.[8] Similarly, a Harvard University Medical School study showed that men with the highest levels of IGF-1 had more than four times the risk of prostate cancer than those with the lowest levels.

In addition, a study by Gregor Furstenberger and Hans-Jorg Senn (2002), at the Center for Tumour Detection, Treatment, and Prevention in St. Gallen, Switzerland, found that IGF-1 is associated with increases in breast, prostate, colorectal, and lung cancers.

One last concern about IGF-1 is that the hormone blocks the body's natural defense mechanisms against early submicroscopic cancers, a natural process known as "apoptosis." This process promotes the growth and invasiveness of early cancers, and also decreases their responsiveness to treatment with chemotherapy. So IGF-1 not only has the potential to make someone more likely to develop cancer, it can also make it more difficult to treat any cancer that may arise.

The increased levels of IGF-1 in rBGH milk are not good for human consumption—at least not past childhood. IGF-1 increases the risks of various types of cancers and can even decrease the effectiveness of conventional cancer treatment. It is worth noting that rBGH milk is banned in Canada, the EU, Australia, New Zealand, and Japan. But it is still on American supermarket shelves, unlabeled.

Benefits of Organic Milk

Organic milk offers benefits beyond just an absence of hormones, antibiotics, and pus. The American Institute of Cancer Research (AICR) reports that milk from grass-fed cows often contains more conjugated linoleic acid (CLA), a type of fat that may protect against cancer and other health problems.[9]

In addition, a clinical report from the American Academy of Pediatrics, published in October 2012 surveyed the scientific literature on organic versus rBGH milk.[10] The researchers point out that much of the difference depends on what the cows eat—which varies by location and by individual farm. However, a number of studies, notes the academy, did show that organic milk has higher concentrations of antioxidants and nutritionally desirable unsaturated fatty acids (conjugated linoleic acid and omega-3 fatty acids) than rBGH milk.

Going Organic

Increasingly, consumers have been responding to all of these concerns by choosing organic milk as the safer alternative. In fact, according to The Hartman Group, organic milk is among the first organic products that consumers buy; they call it a "gateway product." The $4.3 billion organic dairy category has grown by almost 10 percent in 2011 (9.6 percent to be precise), according to the Organic Trade Association. The USDA puts the dollar figure for 2011 at $765 million for sales of organic milk.

On November 9, 2005, *The New York Times* reported that "growth in organic milk is largely driven by continued use of hormones, such as rBGH, and antibiotics in the conventional dairy industry." In 2008, the Nielsen Company reported that "Organics continue to grow and outpace many categories," particularly those marketed to children. Over the past few years, the sale of organic milk has grown by about 20 percent, which is particularly telling at a time when overall milk consumption is dropping by about 10 percent, according to the Hartman Group. The milk market is getting smaller, but, still, people are buying more of the organic variety.

There are more and more producers of organic milk around the country. In 2008, there were more than two thousand farms in the United States producing organic milk. Most of these farms were located in Wisconsin, New York, and Pennsylvania. Though we usually think of California as leading the way in all things organic, fewer than one hundred organic dairy farms were located in California, according to the USDA's Organic Production Survey of 2008.

It helps that it's much easier to locate organic milk. Organic milk originally appeared in supermarkets in 1993, according to the Agricultural Marketing Resource Center, but now is sold all over. Horizon Organic, owned by Dean Foods, is the nation's largest dairy producer, with $192 million annual sales, comprising 55 percent of the market; Organic Valley is the second largest seller; and Stonyfield Farms, owned by Groupe Danone, is the leading French dairy company. Some large grocery store chains, notably Whole Foods Market and Safeway, have their own organic brands. You can even get organic milk at Wal-Mart these days.

Organic milk, though, costs more than regular milk. The USDA, in 2010, determined that organic dairy operating expenses were roughly $4.78 per cwt higher than conventional dairy expenses. There's a good reason the prices are higher: It costs more to produce organic milk than conventional milk. Organic milk production has higher feed costs (food must be organic) and is more labor intensive, according to the USDA.

While feeding cows primarily by pasturing seems as if it would be cheaper than buying feed, the amount of land required to feed a herd of cows is large, so it is actually less expensive to buy organic feed. Partly for this reason, organic dairies are smaller than their conventional counterparts, averaging about 82 cows, as compared with 156 cows on conventional farms. So, when you comparison shop in the supermarket, remember that there are plenty of good reasons for the difference in price tags.

There is another reason why it costs more to produce organic milk than regular milk, of course. Organic dairy farmers don't use those artificial methods of boosting milk production—including Posilac.

The Stonyfield Story

Year Founded: 1983

Products: Stonyfield has three brands. Under the Stonyfield brand, it offers fat-free yogurt, low-fat yogurt, whole milk yogurt, Organic Activia, smoothies, soy yogurt, milk, cream, frozen yogurt, and ice cream. The Yo Babies and Kids brand sells YoBaby Original Yogurt, YoBaby Drinkables, YoToddler Yogurt, YoKids Yogurt, and YoKids Greek Yogurt. Oikos, Stonyfield's organic Greek brand, offers 0 percent fat and 1.5 percent fat Greek yogurt, and frozen Greek yogurt.

Where to Buy: Nationwide

Started as a fund-raising enterprise for the Rural Education Center, a small nonprofit organic farming school in Wilton, New Hampshire, in 1983, Stonyfield Farms has turned into what is arguably the biggest and best-known organic yogurt producer in the country. Their products, which now come from their new plant in Londonderry, New Hampshire, are available in supermarkets and natural food stores coast to coast.

At first, Stonyfield sold just enough yogurt out of its leaky barn to support the farming school. But in 1984, when they were worn out from increased production needs and weary from a night of hand-

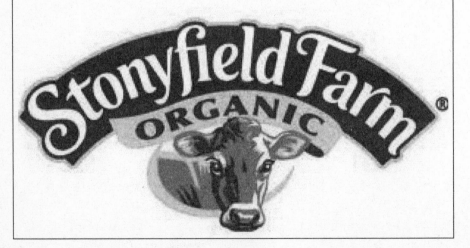

milking after a storm knocked their power out, the founders decided to sell their herd of nineteen cows and purchase milk from local farmers. Thus, a national force was born.

Today, the company retains its commitment to the family farm and to its organic roots. In fact, Stonyfield buys more than three hundred million pounds of organic fruit, organic milk, and other organic ingredients a year, keeping more than two hundred thousand acres of farmland free of pesticides.

On the health front, Stonyfield is dedicated to selling only organic GMO- and rBGH-free food. They say they're the first dairy processor in the nation to pay farmers a premium not to treat cows with rBGH. The company website proudly proclaims, "At Stonyfield, we're committed to producing foods without GMOs as part of our commitment to choosing the best organic ingredients, so we can offer you the healthiest food possible." For more information, see the company website at www.stonyfield.com.

The Nature by Nature Story

Year Founded: 1994

Products: Milk (2 percent, 1 percent, fat-free, buttermilk, chocolate milk); cream (heavy, half and half); whipped cream (with and without brown sugar); 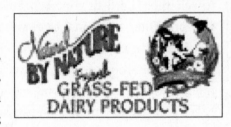 sour cream; French onion dip; Ricotta cheese (regular, lite); and sweet-cream butter (salted, not salted). Nature by Nature is particularly proud of its prize-winning Organic French Onion Dip, which appeared in 2012.

Where to Buy: Whipped cream is distributed nationwide; other products are available on the East Coast.

Located in Lancaster, Pennsylvania, Nature by Nature is a family-owned, organic business, founded by a father and son in their basement in 1984. Ned McArthur had been an organic milk farmer, but quit because he was frustrated by the low prices. But he didn't give up. Ned and his father, Norman, teamed up with four dairy farmers to produce, transport, process, and package organic milk independently.

The plan has worked and today, Nature by Nature has blossomed into a $10 million business. It remains true to its roots and buys all of its milk from other family-owned farms; most of the other farmers are Amish. The cows are all grass-fed. According to the Cornucopia Institute, Nature by Nature cows have plenty of space—about 1.25 cows per acre—and spend between two hundred fifty and three hundred days a year out in the pasture. All products are kosher and gluten-free. In addition, to use sustainable natural resources, Nature by Nature goes green, from its recycled cartons to purchasing all their energy through wind power.

Their mission: "To promote and support organic farming and the sustainable use of our natural resources. To produce foods that benefit consumers and farmers alike. To use the principles of grass-based dairy production as a means to improve the quality of our products, maximize the health of our cows, and protect our watersheds. To make a living for our family, based on these strongly held principles." For more information, see the company website at www.natural-by-nature.com.

The Traders Point Creamery Story

Year Founded: 2003

Products: Creamline milk; aged cheese (Boone County bloomy, Brick Street tomme, riverbend blue, fleur de la terre, farmstead feta); fresh cheese (cottage cheese, fromage blanc); yogurt and Greek yogurt; and ice cream.

Where to Buy: Products are available throughout central Indiana as well as in Illinois, Ohio, Kentucky, Michigan, Minnesota, Missouri, and Wisconsin.

Located in Zionsville, Indiana, Traders Point Creamery is the first USDA-certified organic farm in Indiana; it started in 2003. But it builds on the family's "legacy of sensible, sustainable, low-input agriculture."

The creamery milks between 60 and 90 of its 120 Brown Swiss cows every day throughout the year. Incidentally, the cows spend about 99 percent of their time in the pasture. Traders Point also purchases milk from similarly sized local farms that are also organic and 100 percent grass-fed. The dairy uses no pesticides, herbicides, or synthetic fertilizers, and the cows do not receive antibiotics or synthetic hormones to boost growth. The milk is pasteurized but not homogenized.

The company's mission is to farm in harmony with the land and animals; produce the most nutritious and healthful food possible; encourage education about farming and nutrition; and promote a community of local farm and sustainable farming, reconnecting farmers and consumers. The creamery has a restaurant and the state's only natural, organic, year-round, producer-only market. Speaking to its educational goal, Traders Point Creamery also offers private and self-guided tours for people curious to learn about the organic process from pasture to table. (Private tours can include an optional ice cream tasting.) Visit www.tpforganics.com.

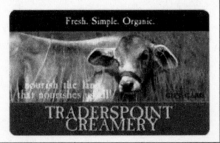

CHAPTER 3

Where's the Beef?

The dairy industry is not the only American industry that uses hormones to boost agricultural production. Hormones have been used for decades in the meat industry to make cows gain more weight, and gain it faster. More weight means more meat and, ultimately, more profit.

The thing is, cows are herbivores by nature. They are meant to eat grass, enjoy the sun, and roam free in pastures. They have a four-chambered stomach designed to convert grass into all the protein and vitamins that they need. The modern livestock farm, though, is not planned with this picture in mind. These days, most cows in the United States are crowded into feedlots and fed mostly corn and other grains. Not the ideal situation for the cows—or for consumers.

Starting with DES

The process of fattening up cows as inexpensively as possible has long been a goal for the beef industry. The precise manner in which the industry has gone about accomplishing this task, however, has evolved over time. Often, it has involved providing something "extra" to the cows.

Early on, farmers gave their cattle a hormone called diethylstilbestrol (DES), one of the first synthetic estrogens. DES was developed at the University of London in 1938. In 1954, the FDA approved oral administration of DES in cattle. Two years later, the FDA approved use of DES implants, according to the American Society of Animal Science.[11]

By that point, DES had already been used in humans, at least in women, for quite a while. Starting in 1938, US physicians prescribed the hormone to women with high-risk pregnancies in order to prevent miscarriages and other pregnancy problems, according to the US Centers for Disease Control and Prevention (CDC). Somewhere between five and ten million pregnant women, and their fetuses, were exposed to the drug. A 1953 study showed that DES didn't actually prevent either miscarriages or premature births.

At about the same time, the controversy over using DES in cattle led to several Congressional hearings on the topic. In 1958, the US Congress passed the Delaney Amendment to the Federal Food, Drug, and Cosmetic Act, banning the deliberate addition of any level of carcinogens into food, based on the assumption that there's no way to set "safe" levels of carcinogens in food. But the USDA and the FDA allowed the meat industry to continue using DES to encourage weight gain in cattle, stating that it did not leave detectable and illegal residues in the meat products. Its use continued to grow nationally.

Physicians continued to prescribe DES for another two decades, until 1971; during this time, as many as four million women took the drug, according to the American Academy of Family Physicians. That year, the FDA advised doctors to stop prescribing DES to pregnant women. Not because of the 1953 study, but rather because of a new study published in the *New England Journal of Medicine* in 1971, led by Arthur L. Herbst at the University of Chicago's Lying In Hospital, that identified the hormone as the cause of a clear cell adenocarcinoma, a rare vaginal cancer.[12] According to the American Academy of Family Physicians, DES was used in some European countries until the early 1980s.

By 1971, DES was being used in 75 percent of US cattle. Researchers found DES residues in cattle and sheep at levels that indicated a connection with the hormone injections. Ultimately, in 1979, DES was banned in US beef. In other words, American women were not permitted to ingest

DES beginning in 1971, but they were allowed to eat its residues, in their dinner food, for an additional eight years.

Moving On to Sex Hormones

When DES was no longer legal for use in US cattle, the United States meat industry looked for other additives to increase beef production. Notably, the industry began using several different natural sex hormones, or a combination of these hormones, implanted into the ears of commercially raised feedlot cattle. The pellets dissolve; there's no need to remove them. Use of these naturally occurring or synthetic sex hormones helps cattle to gain more weight with less feed, making them efficient meat producers.

According to the American Society of Animal Science, the FDA has approved a number of steroid hormone drugs since the 1980s. These include estradiol benzoate/progesterone implants approved for steers in 1956 and for heifers in 1958. Other hormones were developed and approved over time. Specifically, the FDA approved zeranol implants (36 mg) in 1969; silastic estradiol implants in 1982; estradiol benzoate/proges-terone implants (for calves) in 1984; trenbolone acetate implants in 1987; estradiol/trenbolone acetate implants (for steers) in 1991; bovine somato-tropin (for lactating dairy cows) in 1993; estradiol/trenbolone acetate implants (for heifers) in 1994; and estradiol/trenbolone acetate implants (for stocker cattle) in 1996.[13]

Today, the beef industry uses natural estradiol, testosterone, and progesterone as well as synthetic hormones zeranol, trenbolone, and melengesterol to encourage cattle growth. About 90 percent of US cattle are injected with some combination of these hormones.[14] By boosting cattle weight gain, these hormones add about $80 of profit for each animal. These hormones have been prohibited in European beef since 1989, according to Ellin Doyle, PhD, of the Food Research Institute at the University of Wisconsin.[15] The European Union maintains that even exposure to a tiny bit of these hormones carries some level of risk.[16] By contrast, the US government asserts that the levels of these hormones present in American beef are too small to be of any consequence.

However, at least one incident, which took place in Puerto Rico between 1979 and 1981, belies this conclusion. During that period, about three thousand Puerto Rican infants and children developed premature sexual development and ovarian cysts. Researchers discovered that the cysts were caused by hormonal contamination of fresh meat products, which had been contaminated with estrogen residues that were more than ten times the normal. Researchers also found elevated levels of estrogen and zeranol in the blood of these children. In addition, adult women eating the same foods experienced an increase in rates of uterine and ovarian cancers, fibrocystic disease of the breasts, polycystic ovaries, menstrual irregularities, and infertility problems, as described in an article by Leticia M. Diaz in *Boston College Environmental Affairs Law Review* (2000).[17] When the women and children changed their diets to stop eating these meat products, the clinical signs diminished.

Another challenge of industrial farms is that cows are often fed a steady diet of low-dose antibiotics, as we saw in the previous chapter. Farmers and ranchers give cows prophylactic antibiotics, at what is called a "subclinical level" to increase their weight gain and to protect against the mastitis that is frequently caused by the other weight-gain additives fed to the cattle.

This steady diet of antibiotics makes the cattle an ideal breeding ground for the type of drug-resistant bacteria that moves from animals to humans, according to a study by the Translational Genomics Research Institute, led by Lance B. Price, PhD, and published in the journal *Clinical Infectious Diseases* (2011).[18] The study found that nearly half of the meat and poultry samples, 47 percent, were contaminated with *S. aureus*, a bacteria linked to a wide range of human diseases. In addition, more than half of those bacteria, about 52 percent, were resistant to at least three classes of antibiotics, according to the study. "Antibiotics are the most important drugs that we have to treat Staph infections; but when Staph is resistant to three, four, five or even nine different antibiotics—like we saw in this study—that leaves physicians few options," Price explains.[19]

There are many other reasons for antibiotic-resistant organisms, including doctors who overprescribe antibiotics and patients who fail to take their medication correctly. But the FDA has noted that misuse and overuse of these antibiotics in feed animals has contributed as well to the emergence of drug-resistant organisms. The federal agency concludes that:

> In order to minimize the development of antimicrobial resistance, [the] FDA believes that it is important to ensure the judicious use of medically important antimicrobial drugs in animal agriculture. We recommend several steps to accomplish this, including voluntary measures that would limit medically important antimicrobial drugs to uses in food-producing animals that are considered necessary for assuring animal health and that include veterinary oversight or consultation. Such limitations would reduce overall medically important antimicrobial drug use levels, thereby reducing antimicrobial resistance selection pressure, while still maintaining the availability of these drugs for appropriate use.[20]

Feeding Children All-American

As we have seen, the more food is processed, the more room there is for concern about the effects of that processing. When we say "processed," we mean that the meat has been preserved by smoking, curing, or salting, or the addition of chemical preservatives, according to the American Institute for Cancer Research. Processed meats are a good example of the dangers of food processing, and hot dogs are a big concern in this area. They are a mainstay of barbecues and birthday parties. Many kids practically live on hot dogs for a period of time at some point in their childhoods.

The meat industry widely uses nitrates as preservatives in hot dogs (as well as other meat products). When nitrites combine with the amines that are naturally present in meat, they form carcinogenic, N-nitroso compounds. A number of studies show that these compounds cause cancer in animal experiments, particularly cancers of the oral cavity, bladder, esophagus, stomach, and brain.

In 1994, researchers Sara Moir Sarasua and David A. Savitz, PhD, both of the University of North Carolina at Chapel Hill, studied 234 childhood cancer cases in Denver and found a strong association between the consumption of hot dogs and brain cancer, as reported in the *Cancer Causes and Control Journal.* They found that children who were born to mothers who had one or more hot dogs a week during their pregnancies were roughly twice as likely to develop brain tumors. Similarly, children who ate hot dogs at least once a week were also at higher risk of brain cancer. The researchers also found that children who ate hot dogs and took no vitamins (which slow the formation of N-nitroso carcinogens) were more strongly associated with both acute lymphocytic leukemia (ALL) and brain cancer. The authors concluded that:

> The results linking hot dogs and brain tumors (replicating an earlier study) and the apparent synergism between no vitamins and meat consumption suggest a possible adverse effect of dietary nitrites and nitrosamines.[21]

John M. Peters, MD, and colleagues looked at possible causes of the increased risk of leukemia in children from birth to age ten in Los Angeles County between 1980 and 1987. The researchers found that children who ate twelve or more hot dogs a month had approximately nine times the normal risk for developing childhood leukemia. Fathers weren't off the hook, either. There is a strong risk for childhood leukemia for children whose fathers had twelve or more hot dogs a month. In the study published in 1994, the researchers concluded:

> Our results provide evidence for an association between consumption of hot dogs and risk of childhood leukemia. Adjustments for

all factors thought to be potential confounders did not affect these associations. Independent risks were associated with both children's and fathers' consumption. ...The findings, if correct, suggest that reduced consumption of hot dogs could reduce leukemia risks, especially in those consuming the most.[22]

In 2005, Dr. Ute Nöthlings at the Cancer Research Center at the University of Hawaii, analyzed data from a seven-year study of almost two hundred thousand people and found that eating red and processed meats—hot dogs are a prime example of these—was associated with an increased risk of pancreatic cancer. In fact, the people who ate the most of these red and processed foods had a 67 percent higher risk of pancreatic cancer than those who ate little or none, as published in the *Journal of the National Cancer Institute*.[23]

Multiple National Cancer Institute studies had similar findings. For instance, Rashmi Sinha, PhD, at the National Cancer Institute and colleagues found, in 2009, that eating red and processed meat was associated with modest increases in total mortality, cancer mortality, and cardiovascular disease mortality.[24]

Ultimately, the American Institute for Cancer Research (AICR) determined that the link between diets high in red and processed meat and colorectal cancer is convincing. More specifically, every 50-gram serving of processed meat (roughly equivalent to one hot dog) increases the risk of colorectal cancer. To put it another way, people who eat a hot dog every day have a 21 percent higher risk of colorectal cancer than if they never eat hot dogs.[25]

Effects of Radiation

As we have seen, the US beef industry has struggled with contamination for years. Since 2006, it has recalled more than 23 million pounds of beef owing to contamination from Shiga toxin-producing *E. coli* (STEC) bacteria. While this bacteria doesn't hurt the cattle, it might contaminate meat during slaughter, notes the US General Accounting Office (GAO), a federal government research agency. People who eat contaminated meat without properly cooking it are at risk of bloody diarrhea and kidney failure.

The goal of radiation is to keep red meat and poultry from spoiling and to eliminate pathogens such as *E. coli* and *Salmonella*; the USDA compares it to pasteurizing milk. The meat is exposed to radiant energy, usually gamma rays, electron beams, or x-rays. The USDA explains that radiating food does not increase a person's exposure to radiation nor does it make the food itself radioactive.

In 1963, the FDA found beef irradiation to be a safe process. And the federal agency is in good company—the process has also gotten the stamp of approval from the World Health Organization (WHO), the American Medical Association (AMA), the American Dietetic Association, the CDC, the Institute of Food Technologists (IFT), and the American Council on Science and Health (ACSH). According to the CDC, the United States is not alone in radiating its food; France, the Netherlands, Portugal, Israel, Thailand, Russia, China, and South Africa radiate their beef as well.

While it does work for the intended purpose, irradiating meat kills more than just bacteria, parasites, and mold. Radiated beef also loses vitamins B1 (thiamin) and B2 (riboflavin). The USDA explains that the losses are small—and acceptable, because, as USDA chemist Leon Lakritz explains, "We don't eat meal primarily for its vitamin content." Lakritz says, "And cooking can cause greater vitamin loss than irradiation."[26]

However, radiating meat requires medical sterilization facilities, transportation, and additional inspection. Theoretically, these are expenses that could be eliminated by following some basic sanitation rules. Specifically, feedlot pen sanitation, water chlorination, and fly control could drastically reduce cattle infection rates. These rates could be further reduced by feeding hay to the animals seven days prior to slaughter.

Consider Grass-fed Beef

There is a significant difference between grass-fed and corn-fed beef. Grass-fed beef not only lacks hormones and radiation, but it is also healthier in other ways. According to Mayo Clinic cardiologist Martha Grogan on the clinic's website, grass-fed beef offers less total fat, more healthy omega-3 fatty acids, more conjugated linoleic acid (CLA)—which is thought to help prevent cancer and heart disease—and more antioxidant vitamins, such as vitamin E. Research by the Union of Concerned Scientists shows that grass-fed beef also provides high levels of CLA, which has been shown to have positive effects on heart disease, cancer, and the immune system in animal studies.

Cindy A. Daley, PhD, of the California State University–Chico and colleagues have also found supporting evidence. The study, published in the *Nutrition Journal* in 2010, reports that grass-fed beef is

- lower in total fat;
- higher in precursors for vitamins A and E;
- higher in cancer-fighting antioxidants such as glutathione (GT) and superoxide dismutase (SOD);
- influences increased elevated carotenoid content;
- a more desirable SFA lipid profile (which improves cholesterol);
- higher in total omega-3s;
- a better ratio of omega-6 to -3 fatty acids (1.65 vs 4.84);
- higher in CLA (cis-9 trans-11), a potential cancer fighter;
- higher in vaccenic acid, which can be converted to cancer-fighting CLA;
- and lower in saturated fats, which are linked with heart disease.[27]

In short, grass-fed beef offers lower hormone levels and no irradiation. It also provides families with a healthier option for parents and children alike.

Understanding the Labels

Making sense of labels on beef can be confusing, especially if you're not shopping in a small, health food store with a very knowledgeable butcher. It seems as though every producer has its own way of describing the products. The USDA has developed a series of definitions and labels in hopes of bringing some order to this situation. According to the USDA, grass-fed animals get most of their nutrients from grass throughout their life, while organic animals' pasture diet may be supplemented with grain. There's no limit on the use of antibiotics, hormones, or pesticides with either grass-fed or organic beef.

But grass-fed isn't the only label option for beef that has been raised outside of a feedlot. The other possibilities, according to the USDA, are:[1]

- Free-range. This refers to cows that lived in a building, room, or area with unlimited access to food, fresh water, and continuous access to the outdoors during their reproduction cycle. Sometimes, the outdoors area is fenced or netted in, sometimes not. This label is regulated by the USDA.
- Pastured. Usually, this means that cows spend time outside eating grass, but are also fed grain. The term is not regulated by the USDA.
- Grass-finished. The USDA permits organic beef farmers to fatten up a grass-fed herd with corn, soy, or some other grain-based feed, provided that it's organic. A cow that is grass-finished eats grass up until it is led to the slaughterhouse; some farmers think this approach increases the chances of *E. coli* in the beef, according to Rodale.com. Note that not all farmers who feed their cattle exclusively grass use this term.

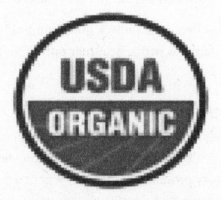

---

[1] There is no standard label for each of these; producers develop their own.

- Cage-free. Here, cows were allowed to freely roam a building, room, or enclosed area with unlimited access to food and fresh water during their reproduction cycle.
- Natural. Beef, poultry, and egg products labeled as "natural" must be "minimally" processed and cannot contain artificial ingredients. But this label doesn't say anything about farm practices, only the processing of meat or eggs.

There are also some labels that don't really provide any information beyond, perhaps, good intentions:

- Pasture-raised. There's no USDA definition here; the meat industry can use it as it wishes, without government regulation.
- Humane. Again, this is an unregulated label.
- No added hormones. Federal regulations have never permitted hormones or steroids in poultry, pork, or goats, so this label simply means the producer followed the basic USDA regulations.

So, read carefully and do your research to be sure of what you are buying and serving to your family.

But the Cost . . .

It's hard to miss the fact that grass-fed beef carries a higher price tag than conventionally raised beef. According to a 2009 article in the *Village Voice*, the price difference is roughly two and a half times. (The paper's reporter paid $9.99 a pound for a Styrofoam-and-plastic wrapped item in the frozen foods section, compared with $26 for a one-pound steak at a specialty store where the butcher was very familiar with the farm where the beef came from).[28] In today's challenging economic times, that minor detail can play a big role in how we feed ourselves and our children.

Grass-fed beef costs more for a variety of reasons, according to the Environmental Working Group (EWG). To begin with, it is unfair to compare the cost of conventionally produced and grass-fed beef because the playing fields aren't level. The federal government subsidizes the cost of corn and soy feed for conventional ranches, but offers no comparable subsidy for grass-fed operations. According to the Physicians Committee for Responsible Medicine, between the years 1997 and 2005, large livestock producers saved an estimated $3.9 billion annually due to the reduced cost of feed containing subsidy-supported corn and soybeans.[29] So the entire country, including vegetarians, is subsidizing the conventional beef industry.

Beyond that, grass-fed cattle is often raised in smaller herds than conventionally fed cattle, and it takes grass-fed cows longer to reach their full weight without growth hormones and antibiotics to speed their growth. Specifically, cows raised on a feedlot can be ready for slaughter at fourteen months, while grass-fed cows aren't ready for a few more months—until they are eighteen to twenty-four months old. So, while the price tag on grass-fed beef is, in fact, much higher than for conventionally grown beef, there are some good reasons for the increase. It is up to us to decide whether the health benefits of grass-fed beef justify the cost for ourselves and our families.

Interest Is Growing

More and more people are deciding that the cost is worth it; they're shopping for beef that was not raised in traditional feedlots. Most of these consumers are motivated more by concern for humane treatment of animals than by concerns for their own health, according to the research by the Leopold Center for Sustainable Agriculture and the Iowa State University Business Analysis Laboratory. These consumers want more information than ever before, notes the Hartman Group. Shoppers are asking about where the meat is coming from; they are increasingly knowledgeable about organic food and look to retailers to give them information that will help them decide which products to put in their grocery baskets.

Whatever the reason, the nontraditional beef business is on the uptick. The organic meat, fish, and poultry market posted tremendous growth in 2011, reaching $538 million in sales. In fact, sales of organic beef alone grew 16.8 percent in 2011, according to the Organic Trade Association (OTA). The greatest portion of the organic meat market was cornered by poultry, which accounted for 61 percent of total organic meat sales. Beef came in second place, with $17 million in new sales, notes the OTA. According to the Food and Marketing Institute, people buy grass-fed beef for five basic reasons. They want:

- better health and treatment of the animal (cited by 44.0 percent of survey participants);
- better nutritional value (43.0 percent);
- better taste (42.0 percent);
- positive, long-term, health effects (41.9 percent);
- and freshness (41.9 percent).

Interestingly, nearly half of American consumers (47 percent) in a recent Whole Foods poll said that they are willing to pay higher for locally produced food; almost a third (32 percent) are willing to pay a surcharge for foods without artificial ingredients, preservatives, or colorings; and almost as many (30 percent) will pay extra for meat with no antibiotics or added growth hormones; and about a quarter (24 percent) will pay more for meats from animals that were raised under humane conditions.

Price, however, continues to restrain sales of natural and organic meat. More than six in ten shoppers (63.0 percent) said they would buy more of these products if they cost less—or at least if the prices were more in line with those of conventionally produced meat—says the Food and Marketing Institute. In other words, most Americans realize the benefits of grass-fed beef, but not everyone is in a financial situation to take advantage of those benefits.

The Brandon Natural Beef Story

Year Founded: 2008.

Products: Steaks, ground beef, and slow-cooked cuts.

Where to Buy: In stores and restaurants in the Bay Area, California; shipped nationally.

Brandon Natural Beef brings grass-fed beef from Colorado's Wet Mountain Valley to Northern California. The mostly Hereford cows graze on alpine grasses, such as Timothy grass, blue grama, red top, and clover and drink from mountain streams; they are 100 percent grass-fed. They live at 8,000 feet above sea level, in the shadow of the Sangre de Cristo Mountains. The animals receive no antibiotics and no hormones and never see a feedlot.

The rancher is Elin Parker Ganschow of Music Meadows Ranch in Westcliff, Colorado, who has been raising cattle all her life, as part of a four-generation family tradition. She selects each individual animal for the Brandon Natural Beef program. In 1968, Elin's parents

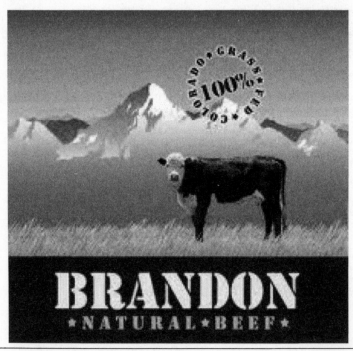

moved her and her five siblings to the ranch. Raised right there, Elin has worked and managed the ranch since she was in high school. And now she is raising four children in the ranching tradition.

The cattle have a relatively low-stress life. They travel ninety minutes to be processed, which means minimal stress on the animal. Cows are slaughtered in small batches of eighty to one hundred cows, which is slower-paced, more humane, and less stressful on the cows than the traditional four-hundred-cows-at-a-time industrial approach. Beef is aged for at least twenty-one days.

The Wet Mountain Valley has a short, intense growing season from September until the end of December; during this time, Brandon Natural Beef sells fresh beef to restaurants. Its retail business is all frozen, and beef is available until they run out. (It has a two-year storage life.) For more information, see the company website at www.brandonnaturalbeef.com.

The KOL Foods Story

Year Founded: 2007

Products: Beef, lamb, chicken, turkey, salmon, and duck.

Where to Buy: Ordered online and shipped, or at a single location in Chicago.

Until July 2007, virtually all kosher meat in the United States was raised conventionally. A kosher consumer who refused to eat unsustainable, caged meat had no choice but to become a vegetarian. What started as Devora Kimelman-Block's quest to find sustainable kosher meat for her family has become a booming business. She established a partnership with a synagogue in Washington, DC, a slaughterhouse, and a local farmer—and, voila, the first glatt kosher (and kosher for Passover), organically raised, local, grass-fed meat available in the United States was produced. Just order online, and it will be shipped to your door.

Kol Foods offers domestic, dry-aged, Black Angus Appalachian Trail Beef, as well as their Grassland Range Beef line. The cows are raised on family farms and are 100 percent grass-fed. They receive no hormones or antibiotics and are not confined to pens or lots. Sustainability is a component of every part of the business. KOL operates out of a LEED-Certified building and uses Energy Star appliances that are wind-powered. One of the slaughterhouses uses biodiesel fuel for its trucks, and the bank is carbon neutral.

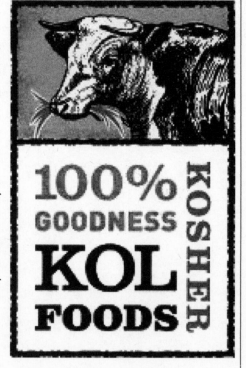

Their vision: "KOL Foods puts glatt kosher meat and ethics on the same plate. Every day, we work to create an honest, transparent food system that treats animals humanely, supports sustainable animal production, treats farmers and workers fairly, and improves the health of families and communities. Our gold standard: animals raised humanely on pasture enjoying their natural diets on sustainable farms, where the environment, health, and concern for the community are paramount. As a values-based business, we produce food that is in harmony with nature, neighbors, and tradition—all the way from farm to fork." For more information, see the company website at www.kolfoods.com.

The Dakota Beef Story

Year Founded: 2007

Products: Beef, boar, goat, lamb, venison, sausage, jerky.

Where to Buy: Certain locations in Arizona, Texas, New York, California, Florida, Georgia, North Carolina, South Carolina, and Virginia.

Located in the high country of eastern Oregon, Dakota Ranch's two ranches provide more than 150,000 acres of native grasses and natural watersheds for the cows. The Angus cattle never receive hormones or antibiotics, eat only certified organic grains and grasses, and have unrestricted outdoor access. In addition, the company also is supplied with organic beef by OBE Beef of Brisbane in Queensland, Australia, which raises its cows in the Australian outback. Dakota Beef's company headquarters are in Howard, South Dakota, where the company also operates its own 33,000-square-foot processing plant, which is certified organic by the USDA.

The website explains, "Dakota Organic Beef provides the purest, most flavorful organic beef around. The only thing you'll taste is simply natural beef, because we never use hormones, antibiotics, or harmful chemicals. And we believe in the importance of sustainable farming, respecting the land and animals, to provide healthy food for your family." For more information, see the company website at www. dakotaorganic.com/dakota-ranch.

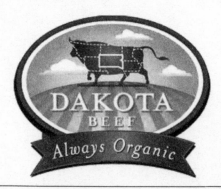

CHAPTER 4
The Dirty Dozen

Probably the number one reason that people buy organic fruits and vegetables rather than conventionally grown is to avoid chowing down on pesticides. After all, pesticides were designed specifically to kill living organisms: insects, plants, fungi, and other "pests." At least in theory, something designed to eliminate organisms can't be good for us.

Studies back up this assessment. According to the Environmental Working Group, pesticides have been linked to a variety of health problems, including brain and nervous system toxicity; cancer; hormone disruption; and skin, eye, and lung irritations. Other research has shown that pesticides are particularly concerning for vulnerable populations—infants and children. We will look at some of these studies below. In short, though, the Organic Center explains that fruits and vegetables account for the majority of pesticide residues and risk in the diet, especially for infants and children.

Even so, probably the first thing to think about is that it's best to do as Mom always said: eat your fruits and vegetables. Basically, the health benefits of a diet full of fruits and vegetables outweigh the risks of pesticide exposure. So, even if you can't afford any organic fruits and vegetables at all, don't decide to avoid the green and leafy altogether. They are always healthier than processed foods or less healthy options.

How to Pick?

As with milk and beef, organic fruits and vegetables are pricier than traditionally grown produce. Some estimates place the cost difference at 20 percent or more higher than traditionally grown produce. Especially these days, when economic times are hard, the higher cost of organic fruits and vegetables can prove a real challenge. So, if you can't buy all organic, if you can only buy some, what should you focus on? The Environmental Working Group (EWG) offers some advice: Avoid the "dirty dozen"—for these fruits and vegetables, go organic. (The Dirty Dozen is more than just a 1960s movie about World War II. It is the EWG's name for those fruits and vegetables that are most likely to be tainted when grown conventionally.) The list:

- peaches
- apples
- sweet bell peppers
- celery
- nectarines
- strawberries
- cherries
- pears
- grapes (imported)
- spinach
- lettuce
- potatoes

In addition, the EWG warns consumers about green beans, kale, and collard greens because, while they do not meet the "dirty dozen" standards, they do display pesticide residues of special concern.

There's another half to EWG's prescription. If you're going to buy conventionally grown fruit, stick with the "clean fifteen," those fruits and vegetables that are the least likely of all conventionally grown items to be tainted with pesticides. For these items, nonorganic is probably fine. The "clean fifteen," as delineated by the EWG, are:

- asparagus
- avocados
- cabbage
- cantaloupe
- corn (both frozen and on the cob)
- eggplant
- grapefruit
- kiwi
- mangoes
- mushrooms
- onions
- pineapples
- sweet peas
- sweet potatoes
- watermelon

These are the safest fruits and vegetables you can buy nonorganic, according to the EWG.

USA, USA

Another suggestion is to buy American, says the Organic Center. Imported produce has much higher levels, in general, of pesticides and pesticide residues. For instance, imported, conventionally grown, sweet bell peppers test at twice as much pesticide and pesticide residue than domestic peppers, while imported nectarines have almost three times as many as their domestically grown counterparts. Imported organic produce, explains the center, is comparable to domestic organic.

How Does EWG Pick the "Dirty Dozen"?

The Environmental Working Group uses data from the US Department of Agriculture and the Food and Drug Administration to evaluate fruits and vegetables for its "dirty dozen" list. (The USDA tests fruit and vegetable samples for dozens of chemicals, sometimes even hundreds of them, according to the EWG.) The EWG then looks at how likely the items are to be consistently contaminated with the most pesticides—both variety and quantity. All fruits and vegetables are washed or peeled, just as you'd do at home.

The Working Group found pesticide residue on 63 percent of all fruits and vegetables tested. Some newspaper and magazine articles have reported that 98 percent of fresh fruits and vegetables have no detectible residues, but EWG explains that this is because the USDA permits some pesticides to be used on certain crops. The list of "acceptable" pesticides varies by crop; what farmers are allowed to use on apples, for instance, is different than what the USDA says is OK to use in growing onions.

Any residues from these "acceptable pesticides" found on the appropriate fruits and vegetables aren't reported by the USDA because they are considered, well, acceptable, according to the Environmental Working Group. On the other hand, the EWG reports all pesticides found on produce, even those that the USDA finds tolerable.

Specifically, the Working Group found that about 98 percent of conventionally grown apples had detectable levels of pesticides, and every single nectarine tested displayed measurable pesticide residues. Beyond that, domestic blueberries had residues of 42 distinct pesticides, grapes had residues from 64 pesticides, and lettuce had 78 different pesticides. Celery and strawberries were found to have 13 different types of pesticides on a single sample, according to the Environmental Working Group.

As for the "clean fifteen," well, more than 90 percent of cabbage, asparagus, sweet peas, eggplant, and sweet potato samples had one or fewer pesticides detected. And no single sample of these fifteen items displayed more than five types of pesticides. Comparatively speaking, that is much better, though it's still not quite 100 percent pesticide-free.

Organic Center Calculations

To get a sense of how many more pesticides are contained in a conventionally grown "dirty dozen" member than in an organic one, consider the Dietary Risk Index (DRI) figures, calculated by the Organic Center, a Washington, DC-based nonprofit focused on research about organic food.

The Center explains that the average American is exposed to between ten and thirteen pesticide residues each day from food, beverages, and drinking water. (Bear in mind that the benefits from avoiding pesticide exposures begin approximately six months before conception and run through young adulthood, and, sometimes, through the entire life span.) The Organic Center looks at pesticide exposures in particular foods, calculating DRI figures. The center looks at both the number of distinct residues, as well as the level of these chemicals. All figures are based on USDA pesticide residue data.

The calculations of these figures are not perfect; they look at individual pesticides but don't take into account that some pesticides work together in harmful ways, causing problems that don't happen when individual pesticides are used by themselves. And these figures are based on the most recent data that the USDA has available, which are not always up to the minute. But they can give you a sense of the comparative safety of organic and conventionally grown fruits and vegetables.

Take lettuce, for example. When tested most recently, conventionally grown lettuce had, on average, residues of 3.9 pesticides in each of 735 samples. Compared with the most recently tested organic lettuce, the conventionally grown vegetable has a DRI that is 120 times higher than the organic. Not an insignificant difference between the two. In general, the Organic Center states, choosing organic fruits and vegetables can cut your intake of pesticides and pesticide residues by 97 percent.

Exposure to Organophosphates

Many insecticides and herbicides contain organophosphate pesticides (also called OP), which are man-made chemicals that the EPA considers toxic to humans. They were originally developed, according to the Public Broadcasting System (PBS), as nerve gas agents for chemical warfar, and they work by paralyzing muscles. People are typically exposed to OP through pesticide residues on the food we eat, according to the CDC. Washing fruits and vegetables before eating helps cut down on consumption of these chemicals, but it doesn't solve the problem completely. Still, researchers maintain, as does the Environmental Working Group, that eating even pesticide-tainted fruits and vegetables is better than avoiding them altogether. We've said it before, but it's important: don't use this information as an excuse to skip your veggies.

Nonetheless, OPs are widespread. Fully 1.2 billion pounds of pesticides were sprayed in both 2000 and in 2001 in the United States, according to the EPA. This little exercise comes with a price tag of about $11 billion each year, the federal government estimates. Around the world, it is estimated that the agricultural industry uses more than 5 billion pounds a year, with an annual cost of about $32 billion, notes the EPA. The catch, according to Walter Crinnion, ND, is that less than 0.01 percent of those pesticides actually make it to the intended pest. So where is that stuff going? This observation raises the question: does eating an organic diet really affect your exposure to OP?

The Organic Center analyzed fruits and vegetables between 1993 and 2006 and found that, over this fourteen-year period, conventionally grown fruit was about 3.2 times more likely than organic fruit to contain a chemical residue, and conventionally grown vegetables were approximately 3.5 times as likely to contain residue as their organic counterparts.

An unusual study led by researcher Chensheng Lu, PhD, at Emory University and colleagues (2006) found that going organic really does cut down on the amount of organophosphate pesticides that you consume. The researchers substituted most of the children's typical food with organic for five consecutive days and collected urine twice daily throughout the experimental period. By comparing the children's urine on organic food with their urine when they were eating traditionally grown produce, the researchers wrote, "In conclusion, we were able to demonstrate that an organic diet provides a dramatic and immediate protective effect against exposures to OP that are commonly used in agricultural production." The study also showed that the children were most likely exposed to these OPs through their diet alone. And if children are exposed to organophosphates through diet, chances are adults are as well.[30]

Even the USDA confirms that organic fruits and vegetables are relatively pesticide-free. According to the Organic Center, approximately 80 percent of organic samples tested by the USDA's "Pesticide Data Program" (PDP) have contained no residues of pesticides. (Incidentally, the CDC states that organophosphates are not likely to build up in animal or plant foods meant for human consumption.)

Effects of These Pesticides

Being exposed to organophosphate pesticides has consequences. Organophosphate pesticides have been shown to damage the nervous system by blocking acetylcholinesterase, an enzyme that stops nerve cells from firing. It can cause a number of other effects in children, notably an increase in the rate of ADHD and of autism, and a lowering of memory and of intellectual capacity as measured by IQ.

Let's start with ADHD. It seems like everyone knows a child—or a handful of children, or a single child who acts like a handful of children— who have been diagnosed with Attention Deficit Hyperactivity Disorder (ADHD). Basically, ADHD is a disorder where people have problems with inattentiveness, overactivity, impulsivity, or a combination of the three. There's a reason the condition seems so prevalent. It is. According to the CDC, parents report that approximately 9.5 percent or 5.4 million children between the ages of four and seventeen have been diagnosed with ADHD, as of 2007. These numbers are increasing by about 3 percent annually. While it's usually children who are diagnosed with ADHD, the problem often persists into adulthood.

Researcher Maryse Bouchard, PhD, and her colleagues looked at more than 1,100 children between the ages of eight and fifteen, of whom 119 were diagnosed with ADHD. The study, which was published in the journal *Pediatrics* in 2010, found that the higher the residue of pesticide in a child's urine, the greater the chance that the child had ADHD.[31]

Pesticides Affect IQ

There's more to worry about than just ADHD. Prenatal exposure to organophosphate pesticides can literally lower a child's IQ. Researchers from the University of California–Berkeley, led by Brenda Eskenazi, PhD, professor of epidemiology and of maternal and child health, found that every tenfold increase in measures of organophosphates detected during a mother's pregnancy corresponded to a 5.5 point drop in overall IQ scores in seven-year-olds.

Another study by Bouchard and colleagues (2011) confirms these results. The researchers studied a group of Latino farm workers' children, testing their urine at six months and at one, two, three and a half, and five years of age and also testing their IQs. The researchers found that the levels of OP in the children's urine were directly correlated with a host of cognitive problems, including reduced IQ points.[32]

Yet another study, this time looking at people living in New York City, also found a connection between levels of OP in urine and cognitive abilities. Since neither these children nor their parents were involved in agricultural work, all the OP in their systems came from the foods they ate, so this study hits home for more of us. Specifically, The Mount Sinai Children's Environmental Health Study (2011) looked at the mother's OP levels during pregnancy and assessed the children at ages twelve to twenty-four months and again at six to nine years of age. The researchers saw evidence of effects beginning when the children were twelve months old and continuing through early childhood.[33]

Pesticides Can Lead to Autism

Exposure to organophosphate pesticides can also lead to autism, which has been on the rise in this country as well. In fact, studies show that the state of California has seen a 600 percent increase in autism diagnoses between 1990 and 2001.[34] The Children's Environmental Health Center

(CEHC) at Mount Sinai School of Medicine developed the list of ten chemicals found in consumer products that are suspected to contribute to autism and learning disabilities. Number four on the list is organophosphate pesticides, followed by organochlorine pesticides. The researchers have also found that organophosphate exposure during pregnancy can impair child cognitive development.[35]

Memory is another area of concern. In 2011, the Columbia Center for Children's Environmental Health, led by Virginia Rauh, PhD, looked at mothers and children in New York City. The researchers measured pesticide exposure through the mothers' umbilical cord blood plasma and then assessed the children's IQs and working memories. They found that for each standard deviation increase in exposure, IQ declined by 1.4 percent and working memory fell by 2.8 percent.[36]

A clinical report from the American Academy of Pediatrics, published in October 2012, looked at the dangers of exposure to pesticides. The academy found that farm workers, who have far more exposure to pesticides than your average supermarket shopper, experienced a number of health problems, including respiratory problems, memory disorders, dermatological conditions, depression, neurological issues (such as Parkinson's Disease), cancer, and problems with pregnancy (miscarriages, birth defects). Infants who had been exposed prenatally often displayed lower birth weight and length and smaller head circumference.[37]

The USDA and FDA both maintain that the residues are within acceptable levels. The FDA states that "parents and caregivers can continue to feed infants their regular baby foods without being concerned about the possible presence of unlawful pesticide chemical residues."[38] But the scientific studies tell a different story. Exposure to organophosphate pesticides, mostly from eating fruit and vegetables that have been treated with OP, can cause a range of neurological disorders.

Benefits of Organic Fruits and Vegetables

The benefits of organic fruits and vegetables are more than just the absence of pesticides. Studies have shown that at least certain organic fruits offer more vitamins and nutrients than their conventionally grown peers.

A study by Washington State University professor John P. Reganold, PhD, and colleagues (2010) found that organically grown strawberries had a longer shelf life and higher antioxidant activity than traditionally grown berries. The researchers also found that organically farmed soils have more total carbon and nitrogen and higher concentrations of micronutrients. In addition, the genes in the soil were better suited than traditional soil genes for several biogeochemical processes, including pesticide degradation.[39]

A second study, by Sho-Ya Wang, PhD, at the State University of New York at Albany, and colleagues (2008) found that blueberries grown from organic culture had significantly higher sugars, malic acid, total phenolics, and antioxidant activity than conventionally grown blueberries. The study looked at blueberries from several organic farms, and while there was some variation from farm to farm, there were still significant differences between conventionally grown and organically grown blueberries.[40]

To get a big-picture idea of the health benefits of organic fruits and vegetables, consider the American Academy of Pediatrics' survey of the scientific literature.[41] The group found that there is a great deal of variation in soils and environments where organic produce is grown, so it is hard to generalize about its benefits. But overall, the academy found that there is more nitrogen in conventionally grown food (lower is better, because nitrogen can increase the risk of gastrointestinal cancer) and higher titratable acidity and phosphorus in organic produce (also a good thing). Most of the studies concluded that organic leafy vegetables (notably spinach, lettuce, and chard) have higher vitamin C concentrations than in the same conventionally produced vegetables. In other words, organic fruits and vegetables offer a plethora of healthy qualities, not just an absence of negative ones.

Baby Food

New parents try their very best to do everything they can to keep their babies safe and happy. They know that infants, whose bodies are still developing, are at the most vulnerable part of their lives. Feeding an infant, especially a first child, can be fraught with anxiety. When do you start serving milk? What about meat? Is there a certain time when you should offer fruits and vegetables? What about organic baby food? It seems as if scientific studies keep coming out and the rules keep changing.

More and more parents are putting their trust in organic baby food. Gerber and Stonyfield have lines of organic baby food, and Abbott Laboratories even offers organic formula, called Similac Organic. Some parents opt for organic baby food to provide environmentally friendly cuisine. Others think it simply tastes better. Still others are concerned that there might be pesticides in conventional baby food. And they would be right, warns the Environmental Working Group.

For the first time ever, the USDA looked at pesticide residues on baby food in 2012 (it has been doing pesticide testing since 1991). They found that green bean baby food tested positive for five pesticides, including two chemicals that the EWG had found in similar concentrations back in 1995, about a decade and a half earlier. Pears were particularly problematic, with 92 percent of all samples tested displaying residues of at least one pesticide, and about a quarter of the samples (26 percent) showing five or more pesticides, including one (iprodione) that is not registered by the FDA for use on pears. This is particularly concerning because, as we have said, babies are considered more, not less, vulnerable than adults to the dangers of pesticides in food. The EPA suggests that infants and children may be more sensitive than adults to pesticides for a few reasons:

- Their internal organs are still growing and maturing. In fact, children's enzymatic, metabolic, and immune systems may provide less natural protection than those of an adult. For instance, because the gastrointestinal tract is still developing, it may be difficult for the body to break pesticides down and eliminate them.

- Infants eat and drink more than adults, in relation to their body weight. After all, their primary project at this stage is to grow. But this increased intake may well increase their exposure to pesticides in food. Beyond that, most babies—and small children, for that matter—eat a narrow range of foods, so they have added exposure to whatever pesticides or other materials are in those foods.

- Also, according to the Institute for Responsible Technology, infants are between three and four times more likely to have food allergies than adults.

The good news is that baby food made of sweet potatoes, a "clean fifteen" food, had virtually no detectable pesticide residues. The "dirty dozen" rule applies to infants, as well as children and adults. The FDA, USDA, and EPA have all issued statements saying that the amount of pesticide residues in baby food is well below the level that would be harmful to infants and children.

History of Pesticide Use

Life on the farm is not as bucolic as Norman Rockwell would have us believe. Farmers have long been engaged in ongoing battles with weeds, insects, and other sorts of pests. But their efforts were met with little success, until pesticides came into their own following World War II, and the introduction of several chemicals, including DDT (dichlorodiphenyl-trichloroethane). DDT was lauded because it was toxic to a wide range of species; it didn't break down in the environment or wash away in the rain (so it didn't need much reapplication); and it was pretty inexpensive. Cheap, simple, and effective—what more could you ask for?

The price, though, came in nonmonetary form. Rachel Carson blew the whistle on human and animal illness and ecological damage in her classic book *Silent Spring*. She outlined how DDT affected fish and crabs, as well as unwanted insects. Some of the pests became genetically resistant to pesticides, and researchers began noticing pesticide residues in unexpected places.

When the EPA was created in 1970, it took on the task of overhauling pesticide regulation, in light of the new findings. Under the Federal Environmental Pesticides Control Act (FEPCA), pesticide manufacturers had to conduct tests to demonstrate that their products did not have "unreasonable adverse effects" on human health or the environment. The EPA could choose not to register any product that it decided was unsafe for human consumption. As a result, the EPA pulled DDT off the market in 1972, though some developing countries continued to use it for a number of years after that.

In 1996, Congress passed the Food Quality Protection Act, which gave the EPA the job of completely overhauling the US pesticide and food safety laws. The Act changed the EPA's safety standards, especially in regard to infants and children. Thus far, the EPA has banned use of 6,224 pesticides, including some that are considered to pose the greatest risks to children.[42] For instance, the EPA has:

- cancelled some uses of methyl parathion, a compound considered one of the most toxic organophosphates;[43]
- phased out most nonagricultural uses of chlorpyrifos (Dursban) and restricted its use on tomatoes and apples;[44]
- barred diazinon use on about twenty different crops, primarily vegetables;[45]
- barred the neurotoxic pesticide carbofuran for all food crops at the end of 2009.[46]

But we still have a way to go—and organophosphate pesticides are ripe for reform.

In the Market

Organic fruits and vegetables are the most commonly purchased organic food items in the United States, according to the Organic Trade Association, accounting for approximately 40 percent of all organic food sales in 2011; that is a big increase from the 2009 figure, which was 11.8 percent.

Most of the sales are in fresh produce (92.9 percent), with a little bit of frozen (3.0 percent) and canned (2.7 percent) organic fruits and vegetables being sold as well. Apples—one of the Environmental Working Group's "dirty dozen"—were the biggest seller among organic fruits, while packaged salad led the way among vegetables. In 2011, organic vegetables outsold organic fruits at more than two to one, according to the USDA. Overall, organic vegetable sales amounted to $1.1 billion, while fruits sold at $494.8 million. The top-selling fruits were (of course) apples ($122.2 million of the total) and grapes ($160.6 million).

Let's take a look at Washington State, the country's leading producer of conventionally grown and organic apples, pears, and cherries. In 2010, for instance, the western state had 20,658 acres of certified organic tree fruit. Clearly, public interest in organic fruit trees is increasing; in 1998, organic apples represented 1 percent of the total acres planted with apples and organic pears, and represented only 2 percent of the total acres for pears. But by 2010, according to the Center for Sustaining Agriculture and Natural Resources at Washington State University, organic apples were a full 10 percent of total apple acreage planted. Similarly, organic pears sales rose 50 percent between 2005 and 2010. Americans are noticing the importance of organic fruits and vegetables to lifelong health. And we're "voting" with our pocketbooks—and with our stomachs.

After the world has devoted so much time and energy into developing ways to add hormones and organophosphates to our fruits and vegetables, it is time to reverse the trend. We need to focus our attention on developing new ways to improve the healthfulness of our foods. Going organic, at least partway, is the best way to accomplish this goal. (See chapter 7: Avoiding GMOs, page 97, for suggestions.)

The Swanton Berry Farm Story

Year Founded: 1983

Products: Strawberries, olallieberries, blackberries, tayberries, loganberries, boysenberries, kiwis, artichokes, broccoli, cauliflower, pumpkins, peas, Brussel sprouts, and celery. There are also a variety of homemade jams.

Where to Buy: Nine farmers' markets in the San Francisco area.

Swanton Berry Farm was founded by two veteran cooperative farmworkers. Based in Davenport, California, they tried organic farming when everyone told them it couldn't be done. They rented four acres of land, bought an old tractor, and planted the entire area with strawberries. In 1987, the farm was certified by California Certified Organic Farmers, becoming the first organic strawberry farm in the state. The following year, Swanton Berry Farm was the first organic farm to sign a contract with the United Farm Workers, AFL-CIO.

These days, the farm grows two varieties of strawberries, the Chandler and the Seascape, and they try other varieties as well, in addition to a wide variety of other fruits and vegetables. Not only have the number of crops grown, but, in 2011, Swanton Berry Farm rented two hundred acres in five different locations. Swanton Berry Farm does it in the conscientious way, using organic farming methods and 100 percent union labor.

The farm is committed to sustainability and, in 2002, won the EPA Stratospheric Ozone Protection Award for developing a technology to harvest strawberries without using methyl bromide, a major contributor to depletion of the ozone layer. On the farm's website, Swanton Berry Farm writes, "We see ourselves as a tiny part of a huge system of food producers and food 'eaters' that is just beginning to develop its own 'consciousness.'" For more information, see the company website at www.swantonberryfarm.com.

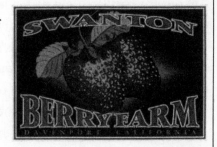

The Hoch Orchard and Gardens Story

Founded: 1992

Products: Apples, wine grapes, raspberries, strawberries, raspberries, blueberries, blackberries, apricots, cherries, apricots, peaches.

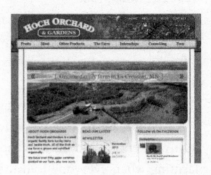

Available: Use order form at www.hochorchard.com.

Based in La Crescent, Minnesota, Hoch Orchard and Gardens is a small, family-owned organic farm run by Harry and Jackie Hoch, a farm with a long history. The orchard's first trees were planted in the mid-1940s, though there are only a handful of these old trees left on the farm today. Most of the ten thousand trees now on the thirty-acre farm have been planted in the past ten years.

Originally a conventional farm, Hoch Orchard and Gardens completed its transition in 2010, and the whole farm became certified organic. Recently the farm started using high-tunnel greenhouses to extend the growing season. The tunnels help berries start ripening earlier and produce later in the fall. The first tunnel houses strawberries, as well as black, purple, red, and yellow raspberries, and a few blackberry bushes. The second tunnel is devoted to strawberries, blackberries, and sweet cherry trees. The Hoch extended family is involved in farming as well.

To develop a truly sustainable system, the Hoch Orchard and Gardens is also incorporating animals into its farm. The farm raises hogs, chickens, ducks, and geese. The plan is for these animals to help reduce the amount of organic fertilizers and pesticides at the farm. The website itself says: "Our little farm is a vertically integrated food production system. We only sell fruit that we grow. This way, you know where the food came from, who actually produced it, and how it was produced. We do not buy fruit from other farmers and put our label on it. If it says Hoch Orchard and Gardens on the bag, the fruit inside was grown by us." For more information, see the company website at www.hochorchard.com.

The Jerzy Boyz Farm Story

Founded: 1989

Products: Pears and apples

Available: Order by mail at www.jerzyboyz.com/jerzybrochure. htm.

A Big Apple girl and a Jersey boy arrived in Washington State and, after working twenty years farming apples for North Central Washington growers, started their own orchard. In 1989, Wynne Weinreb and Scott Beaton purchased a piece of virgin land a few miles north of Lake Chelan in the foothills of the Cascade Mountains, overlooking the Columbia River. They became interested in organic food in the 1970s, when Wynne began eating organic cheese, fruits, vegetables, and whole grains. They started growing their own organic gardens in 1980.

Today, the five-acre orchard, planted with pear and apple trees, uses hand-thinning instead of chemical thinning; manual weed

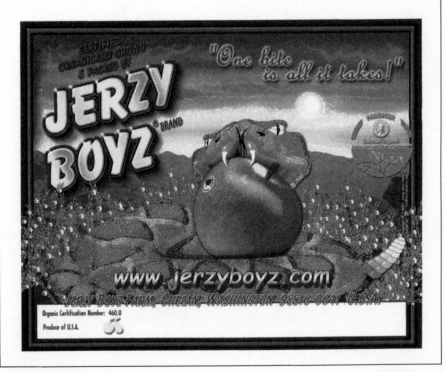

control instead of chemical herbicides; and hand removal of unwanted pests. It also uses customized composts, mineral applications, and foliar feedings. The Jerzy Boyz have used a variety of cover crops, rather than grass, and they prefer red clover. They find that red clover offers a nice habitat for beneficial insects, helps create a lush environment that fruit trees thrive in, and adds a lot of nitrogen to the soil when it is mowed. The Boyz make their own compost and brew it in 400-gallon tanks with water and nutrients. The website explains: "Organic farming is a lot of fun in some ways—you get to grow and eat your own healthy fruit, you get to test new varieties and work with composting, which is really a lot of fun, and you get to share your healthful product with people." For more information, see the company website at www.jerzyboyz.com.

CHAPTER 5

Going Against the Grain: Corn and Soybeans

Corn and soybeans are two of the most popular, versatile, and sneaky foods in the world. Corn is actually the most produced grain around the globe, providing about 21 percent of human nutrition, according to the Whole Grains Council. And soybeans, notes the USDA, are the second-most-planted field crop in the United States after corn, with 77.5 million acres planted in 2009.

The origin of corn was a puzzle for years. It doesn't actually grow wild anywhere at this point, so its beginnings are hard to track down. A team of botanists, geneticists, and archaeologists managed to trace it to the tropical Central Balsas River Valley in Mexico, determining that it was domesticated about nine thousand years ago. The other area of confusion is corn's classification: according to the Whole Grains Council, fresh corn is usually classified as a vegetable, and dried corn (including popcorn) is a grain.

The reason corn is sneaky? You may think it just comes into your life as a slice of cornbread or a butter-and-salt-slathered side dish. But it's an ingredient in about three thousand products including ethanol, cosmetics, ink, glue, laundry starch, medicines, and fabrics. So, if you're driving a car, sipping a soda, and digging into a bag of chips, chances are you're surrounded by corn.

The soybean is a legume that hails from East Asia. The United Nations Food and Agricultural Organization (FAO) classifies it as an oilseed. Soybeans are a widespread source of protein for animals, as well as humans. And they're efficient protein producers; if you want to get the maximum amount of protein per cultivated acre, you'd plant soybeans, notes the National Soybean Research Laboratory.

In addition to protein, soybeans provide oil and appear in a wide variety of processed foods including, oddly, fertilizer. But most of the soybean produced in this country becomes soybean meal and vegetable oil. The United States is both the world's biggest producer of soybeans— and the world's largest consumer of them, according to Spectrum Commodities.[47]

Soybeans have a split personality, just as corn. They can be broadly classified as "vegetable" (garden) or "field" (oil) types. Vegetable types of soybeans cook more easily, have a mild, nutty flavor, better texture, are larger in size, higher in protein, and lower in oil than field types. They can become soy milk, tofu, plastics, inks, lubricants, and diesel fuels, according to the United Soybean Board. They are also common in baby formula. Probably the strangest use was developed by Henry Ford, who built a car with a body made of soybeans.

Monsanto's Roundup

In 1984, Monsanto Corporation introduced Roundup, a broad-spectrum herbicide made of glyphosate designed to target broadleaf and cereal leaf weeds; it is a type of organophosphate. It is designed, Monsanto notes on

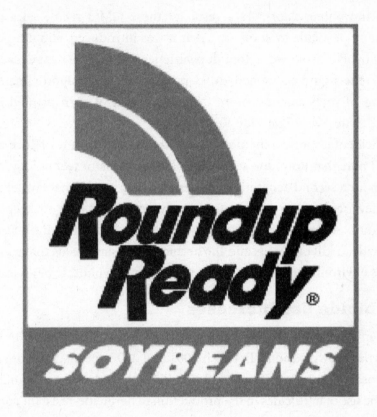

its website, to be absorbed throughout the plant's tissues. The herbicide then inhibits the activity of EPSP synthate, an enzyme essential for plant life. Roundup's effectiveness made it popular within the agricultural community.

Roundup pesticide became even more popular in 1996. That's the year that Monsanto began to introduce Roundup Ready crops, which were genetically modified to be resistant to the aforementioned herbicide. So, a farmer could plant Roundup crops, spray them with Roundup pesticide, and know that the crops would be untouched by the pesticide.

The first Roundup Ready crop was soybeans, followed by alfalfa, corn, cotton, canola, and sugar beets. As with Roundup Ready corn, these other Roundup Ready plants can tolerate the glyphosate pesticide, so farmers who use these crops also use Roundup pesticide to eliminate weeds and other unwanted plants. As a result of these GMO seeds, sales of the Roundup pesticide took off. The year it was introduced, about 8 percent of all soybeans sold were Roundup varieties. Within the next decade and a half, the figure ballooned to 93 percent. In 2012, approximately 95 percent of soybeans and more than 85 percent of corn planted in the United States were Roundup Ready.

Incidentally, researchers at the Massachusetts Institute of Technology (MIT) note that Roundup seeds also have "terminator technology." Seeds grown for a second generation are sterile, which means that farmers must buy new seeds from Monsanto every year if they wish to keep using Roundup. So every year, farmers write huge checks to Monsanto—for herbicide to kill off weeds and the herbicide-resistant seeds that can grow in this environment—all in order to perpetrate glyphosate pesticide.

Herbicide Use Increases

Since it was introduced, Roundup pesticide use on these Roundup Ready crops has grown steadily. Between 2001 and 2007, for instance, use of the glyphosate herbicide doubled to 185 million pounds. No one anticipated that the use of herbicides in the production of herbicide-resistant corn and soybeans would increase use of pesticides; in fact, part of the point of genetically modified crops was to cut down on the amount of pesticide used.

But that's exactly what Charles Benbrook, PhD, Chief Scientist at the Center for Sustaining Agriculture and Natural Resources at Washington State University, found. His analysis showed that glyphosate-tolerant crops worked very well for a few years. Then some weeds, including horseweed, giant ragweed, and pigweed, developed a resistance to Roundup, thereby earning the title "superweeds." These superweeds are now taking over millions of hectares of farmland in the United States and around the world. According to an article in *Natural Society Magazine*, they cover 4.5 million hectares in the United States and an estimated 120 million hectares worldwide.[48] Farmers have responded by increasing their use of the herbicide, which, of course, may well lead to even more build-up of herbicide resistance.[49]

Dangers of Glyphosate

The concern is not just that farmers are needing to use more and more glyphosates—after all, if glyphosates were perfectly safe, who would care? The question is: are they?

Herbicides are used specifically to kill off weeds and other pests, so it is not surprising that they harm plants. But it *is* surprising to find that herbicides can affect amphibians. A study performed by Rick A. Relyea, PhD, Director of the Pymatuning Laboratory of Ecology at the University of Pittsburgh, did a study published in 2005 that demonstrated that Roundup herbicide completely eliminated two species of tadpoles, leopard frogs, and gray tree frogs, and nearly exterminated a third species, the wood frog; in fact, the wood frogs were left at 2 percent of their former population. All in all, this led to a 70 percent decline in the species richness of tadpoles.[50] Frogs weren't pinpointed as targets for the pesticide; this finding suggests that glyphosate can affect organisms beyond the pests they are intended to kill.

A second study, published in the journal *Chemical Research in Toxicology* in 2010 by Alejandra Paganelli and colleagues at the Universidad Buenos Aires, found that chicken embryos treated with glyphosate-based herbicides (Roundup was not specified in the study) were born with deformities and neurological problems; the researchers determined that it was the glyphosate alone that caused these effects.[51]

It is important to realize that Roundup is not pure glyphosate. It also contains a "surfactant" designed to help the chemicals penetrate the plant leaves; the surfactant is not supposed to be dangerous in itself—its purpose is only to help the glyphosate kill pests more effectively. But studies have shown that the "inert" ingredients in herbicides can also be harmful to humans.

These ingredients are rarely identified on product labels because they are often considered "proprietary," and as the pesticide mixtures become more and more complicated, it is apparent that the pesticide formulations act differently than individual, active ingredients alone. This sentiment has been echoed by the National Research Council, the

Agency for Toxic Substances and Disease Registry, and the American Medical Association.[52]

There's a scientific phenomenon of gene flow, where genes transfer from one population to another, say from a GMO plant to a plant that wasn't originally genetically modified. It's a natural phenomenon and occurs with a range of species and can happen via pollen and seed. Carol Mallory-Smith, PhD, at Oregon State University and colleagues have found that genes can "flow" from glyphosate-resistant crops to others, adding to the challenge of weed management and enabling glyphosate-resistant weeds to take over ever more acreage.[53] Presumably, this process would lead to even more use of herbicides.

Glyphosate-resistant Alternatives

An alternative to using more and more glyphosate, of course, is to switch to a different herbicide. Bayer CropScience has responded to the challenge with a series of glyfosinate-ammonium-based herbicides that work on glyphosate-resistant weeds: they are Liberty, Basta, Rely, Finale, and Ignite. The Liberty herbicide offers the full package, with Liberty-resistant crops available as well: LibertyLink soybeans, corn, cotton, and canola. Just as with Roundup Ready crops, Bayer CropScience sells both a challenge—an herbicide that will kill wanted crops as well as weeds—and its solution, glyfosinate-resistant strains of the crops.

Chemical manufacturers are also turning to older pesticides to try to combat glyphosate-resistant weeds. One of the most popular is 2,4-Dichlorophenoxyacetic acid, or 2,4-D, a herbicide/pesticide that was developed during World War II and is a major ingredient in Agent Orange, a defoliant used in the Vietnam War; the Vietnamese government estimates that about four hundred thousand people were killed or maimed, and roughly five hundred thousand children were born with birth defects as a result of Agent Orange. A common, systemic pesticide/herbicide used to control broadleaf weeds, 2,4-Dichlorophenoxyacetic acid is, according to the EPA, the main ingredient in more than fifteen hundred pesticide and herbicide products. While it may be an older pesticide, 2,4-D still does the job.

Bt Corn

One of the relatively new options in the world of pesticides is *Bacillus thuringiensis* plant-pesticides, also called Bt. These plants themselves function as pesticides. They are resistant to glyphosate and have an additional self-defense mechanism—they exude the bacterial Bt toxin, which is poisonous to certain types of insects, including European corn borers.

There are several types of Bt corn. Some target above-ground pests, while others focus on those in the soil. There are currently eight registered *Bacillus thuringiensis* (Bt) plant-pesticides, one each for Bt potatoes, Bt cotton, and Bt popcorn, and five for Bt field corn, according to the EPA.

In 1999, John Losey at Cornell University found that Bt was dangerous for monarch butterflies, often considered a bellwether for the safety of other animals. In a laboratory test, the butterflies were fed milkweed leaves dusted with transformed pollen from a Bt Corn hybrid. They ate less than those that weren't fed the Bt and suffered a higher mortality rate—in fact, nearly half of the "test" butterflies died.[54] When the study was assessed again, three years later, researchers from the Pew Initiative on Food and Biotechnology found that the risks to monarch butterflies was fairly small, if only because the larvae are only exposed to low levels of Bt corn pollen in the "real world." The long-term effects, though, are still uncertain, according to the Pew Trusts.[55]

The Politics of Corn and Soybeans

The prominent role that GMOs play in today's food markets stems from the Great Depression of almost a century ago. The then-unprecedented economic crisis hit the farm sector hardest. The prices that farmers got for their goods in the market fell by more than 50 percent, while the prices of goods and services that farmers had to buy declined by 32 percent, leaving farmers in a hole, according to the USDA.[56]

In response, the federal government put into place a series of interrelated laws designed to maintain the American food supply; the laws affected a variety of crops, including corn. Basically, in order for the government to control both prices to the consumer and the amount of product available, the government agreed to, essentially, pay farmers *not* to work all their land; specifically, corn growers in 1933 were to plant at least 20 percent less than their average acreage over the previous two years. In 1940, price supports were implemented for various crops, including corn, to make sure farmers didn't lose money by planting fewer crops. At the same time, the USDA was developing programs to dispose of the surplus food, while raising the nutritional level of low-income consumers. The government instituted three national programs: school lunch, low-cost milk, and food stamps. These programs took care of much of the surplus food.

In the 1960s, the combination of fertilizers, pesticides, farm machinery, and improved seeds led farmers to record production; corn production, for instance, grew 65 percent, and in 1960, there was a surplus of about 1.8 billion bushels (a bushel of corn is equivalent to eight "dry" gallons). By 1970, world crop shortages had the entire globe turning to the United States, and while US corn production grew about 25 percent between the late 1960s and 1973, by 1973, the government surplus had shrunk to zero. Crop supports were readjusted yet again. It was the same old problem: American farmers could produce much more corn (and other crops) than was needed in the United States or around the world.

Since the 1970s, according to the Physicians Committee for Responsible Medicine, US agricultural policies have increasingly encouraged the overproduction of agricultural commodities, including corn and soybeans, resulting in a glut of crops. The overabundance of cheap feed crops encouraged the growth of large factory farms. The Committee states that corn and soybeans together have received more than $96 billion in subsidies between 1995 and 2010.[57]

At the same time, the Energy Policy Act of 2005 mandated use of renewable fuels in gasoline. These days, most gasoline contains a certain amount of biofuel—usually ethanol, which is made from fermenting and distilling the simple sugars in corn—that must be mixed with gasoline sold in the United States. The Act required that 4 billion gallons of biofuel be used by 2006, 6.1 billion gallons by 2009, and 7.5 billion gallons by

2012. Fuel ethanol reduces the carbon monoxide content of engine exhaust and reduces engine knock.[58]

The Energy Independence and Security Act of 2007 extended the law so that there would be a requirement to mix 36 billion gallons of biofuel in with gasoline by 2022. This demand for ethanol, notes the USDA, has pushed up corn prices and encouraged farmers to devote more land to growing corn. Specifically, the percentage of corn used for fuel alcohol grew from less than 1 percent of total US domestic corn use in 1980–1981 to almost 25 percent in 2007–2008. Currently, the federal government pays about $20 billion a year to farmers in the form of farm subsidies. When it comes to subsidy payments, corn leads the way. In 2004, the USDA estimates that about 35 percent of subsidies went to corn and 7.6 percent went to soybean subsidies.

Advantages to Earth and Workers of Organic Farming

Organic farming produces the same yields of corn and soybeans as conventional farming, according to a 2005 study by Cornell University professor David Pimentel. But some of the costs are lower—notably organic farming uses 30 percent less energy as well as less water, and, of course, no pesticides. The twenty-two-year study also found that during the drought years, 1988 to 1998, organic corn yields were 22 percent higher than in the conventional fields. In addition, organic farming reduced local and regional groundwater pollution by not applying agricultural chemicals.[59]

There are several other advantages to organic farming over conventional farming, according to the Rodale Institute, a nonprofit organization dedicated to spreading the word about organic farming. The institute says that organic farming is easier on the soil, causing less erosion and maintaining the soil quality; in fact, it builds up the soil. Organic farming uses 45 percent less energy and produces 40 percent less greenhouse gases than conventional farming. In addition, the Rodale Institute notes, organic corn and soybean crops tolerate much higher levels of weed competition than their conventional counterparts, producing equivalent yields.[60]

The issues of cost aren't just about organic crops. A 2012 study by the Union of Concerned Scientists found that the organic dairy sector provides more economic opportunity and generates more jobs in rural areas than conventional dairy farms. Looking at financial data from Vermont and Minnesota, two major milk-producing states, researchers found that increases in dairy sales from organic dairy farms contributed more to the state in terms of employment, labor income, and gross state product than similar increases in conventional dairies.[61]

Why Do Organic Foods Cost More?

For starters, according to organic.org, organic farmers don't receive the same subsidies as conventional farmers. Nor do the price tags on conventionally produced foods include a number of other federal (taxpayer) subsidies, such as the cost of cleaning up polluted water and remediating land contaminated with pesticides. The Rodale Institute points out that a proper accounting of the societal costs of conventional farming would also consider that fertilizer run-off damages fisheries, as well as the increased health risks that agricultural workers and their communities experience due to exposure to pesticides and antibiotic-resistant bacteria.

In addition, organically produced foods, notes the Organic Farming Research Foundation, must meet stricter government regulations and require much more intensive management and labor than their conventionally grown counterparts; the labor costs are often, though not always, more expensive than the cost of chemicals on traditional farms. The research foundation also notes that there is evidence that if all the indirect costs of conventional food were factored into its price tag, it would cost about the same as the current cost of organic food.

Some studies show that even with these additional challenges, organic soybeans can still end up with higher profits than conventionally grown soybeans. In Minnesota, organic soybean yields in 2008 averaged 18 bushels per acre, compared to 40 bushels per acre for conventional beans, according to the University of Minnesota's FinBin, a database of farm financial performance, as quoted in *Corn and Soy Bean Digest*.[62] Gross revenues for organic beans averaged $538 an acre, and expenses averaged about $355 per acre. By comparison, gross revenues on conventional beans averaged $432 for each acre, and expenses averaged $332 per acre. While the profit margins on both organic and conventional soybeans are tight, organic soybeans returned about $80 per acre more than conventional beans in 2008.

The Market

Despite the fact that there are some pricing issues, production for both organic corn and organic soybeans is increasing. That trend is expected to continue. Take a look at corn. In 1995, for instance, organic grains grew on 32,650 acres, according to the Agricultural Marketing Resource Center, a collaborative project of the USDA and Iowa State University; this figure reached 194,637 in 2008.[63] Most production happens in Wisconsin, Minnesota, Iowa, Michigan, and New York, but a total of thirty-seven states grow organic corn. The majority went to feed livestock and the rest for us humans. More than 90 percent of this organic corn stayed in the United States. The USDA notes that organic corn sales hit $101.5 million in 2011.

Organic soybean production has grown faster than any other consumer food group, according to the Agricultural Marketing Resource Center (1995), though soybean production dropped 8 percent between 2010 and 2011, falling to about 3.1 billion bushels. Just as with corn, the top producers are Iowa and Illinois, followed by Minnesota and Nebraska. According to the Center, experts estimate that US soybean production hit $2.97 billion in 2012; but, the Center notes, this is only 1 percent of total soybean production in the United States. Organic is gaining ground in the soybean arena, but it still has a way to go.

The Eden Foods Story

Year Founded: 1968

Products: Organic beans canned and dry, organic condiments and sweeteners, organic chili, organic sauces and butters, organic soy, organic fruit juices, traditional Japanese foods, organic oils and vinegars, organic pasta, organic rice and beans, sea vegetables, organic spices and herbs, organic supplements and concentrates, organic teas, organic tomatoes, organic sauerkraut, organic dried fruits and nuts, and organic beans.

Where to Buy: Natural food stores, co-ops, supermarkets nationwide—and on the web.

The oldest natural and organic food company in North America, Eden Foods was born in Ann Arbor, Michigan, in the late 1960s and has been owned and operated independently for more than four decades. It started as a co-op and has evolved into a natural food store offering whole grains, beans, soy foods, cereals, vegetable oils, seed oils, and seed and nut butters. These days, it also offers a cafeteria, bakery, and a book section. But it still buys most of its food from local farmers, except (of course) for the extra virgin olive oil (from Spain), high-altitude white and red quinoa (from the Andes Mountains), chamomile (from Egypt), and traditional Japanese foods from the Far East.

In 1972, Eden established relationships with Japanese traditional food makers and began to import sea vegetables, teas, miso, shoyu, umeboshi plums, kuzu root stach, rice vinegar, rice bran pickles, and mirin to stock its very first warehouse.

Eden Foods do not carry the USDA Organic seal, but maintain that their products meet or exceed all USDA organic standards. The Cornucopia Institute says, "Based on our follow-up research, we have no reason to question their claim that all soybeans used in their EdenSoy products come from American farmers with whom they have long-term and stable relationships." Please note that Eden Foods does sell four products containing non-US-grown soybeans: natto miso, freeze-dried tofu, tekka tofu, tekka sauce, and ponzu sauce.

The company goals are to: "provide the highest quality, life-supporting food and accurate information about them, their uses, and benefits; to maintain a healthy, respectful, challenging and rewarding environment for employees; to cultivate sound relationships with other organizations and individuals who are like-minded and involved in like pursuits; to cultivate adaptability to change in economic, social, and environmental conditions, to allow Eden the opportunity to survive long-term; to have a strong, positive impact on farming practices and food-processing techniques used throughout the world; and to contribute to peaceful evolution on earth." For more information, see the company website at www.edenfoods.com.

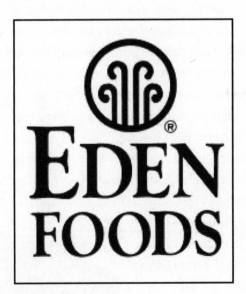

The FarmSoy Company Story

Year Founded: FarmSoy Company has been making soymilk and tofu since the early 1970s, and the products have been certified organic since 1992.

Products: Tofu and dairy-free soy yogurt.

Where to Buy: Locally and Fresh Market stores nationwide.

The Summertown, Tennessee, institution was originally called the Farm Soy Dairy and was started, in the early 1970s, to diversify the food options of the vegan Farm Community during its early communal period. The community changed and so did the dairy, becoming a business, with the name FarmSoy Company, in 1983.

The current owners bought the company in 1991, and it has been certified organic since 1992. The company maintains personal relationships with the farmers in Missouri and Illinois who grow the USDA-certified organic soybeans the company uses. FarmSoy then uses the community's well water (which is tested regularly) and calcium sulfate to coagulate the soymilk and form tofu, a process approved by the National Organic Standards Board. All manufacturing is done in-house. In addition to tofu, FarmSoy offers a high protein, dairy-free, sugar-free, plain soy yogurt, called Soygurt. The product contains no thickeners or additives and can be used as a substitute for buttermilk in baking.

The website explains: "FarmSoy tofu is made by craftsmen who love to eat tofu and take pride in creating a firm, yet creamy tofu to satisfy your palate. The large corporate brands of tofu are made entirely by machine, and you can tell the difference! We also like to use the highest quality of only certain varieties of soybeans." For more information, see the company website at www.farmsoy.com.

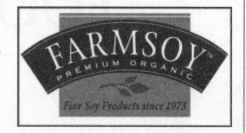

The Lakeview Organic Grain Story

Year Founded: 2001

Products: Certified organic feed grains (corn, roasted soybeans, peas, soybean meal, flax meal, barley, oats, wheat, and sunflower meal), bagged feed, approved supplements, and organic crop seeds (hybrid and OP corn, soybeans, barley, oats, wheat, rye, buckwheat, spelt, triticale, field peas, winter peas, clover, alfalfa, Timothy, and other pasture/cover crop grasses and legumes).

Where to Buy: Bulk feed delivered in New York State and northern Pennsylvania; shipped throughout the Northeastern United States.

Mary-Howell and Klass Martens started out in agribusiness, but became worried that Klass's perennially aching head and queasy stomach stemmed from using pesticides. They decided to convert their Penn Yan, New York, farm to organic in 1993. Three years later, three organic dairy farmers approached Mary-Howell and Klaas Martens and asked if they could start making organic cow feed. Pretty soon, they had 150 organic dairy farmer customers. They purchased the Agway Feed Mill in Penn Yan and converted it into an organic feed mill, which is now called Lakeview Organic Grain.

These days, Mary-Howell and Klass Martens farm 1400 acres of organic corn, soybeans, small grains (wheat, spelt, barley, oats, and triticale), field peas, winter peas, dark red kidney beans, and edamame soybean. They also raise organic cows, pigs, chickens, and most importantly, three children, all involved in farmwork.

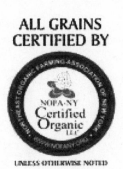

ALL GRAINS
CERTIFIED BY

NOFA-NY
Certified
Organic
LLC

UNLESS OTHERWISE NOTED

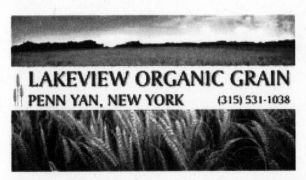

LAKEVIEW ORGANIC GRAIN
PENN YAN, NEW YORK   (315) 531-1038

Lakeview Organic Grain emphasizes the comfort of the animals: comfortable stalls, dry bedding, good ventilation in the barn, plenty of water for every animal, walkable flooring free of mud or ice, and sufficient forage and silage, with particles big enough for proper chewing and ruminating (chewing the cud).

As Mary-Howell writes, "Too often we view the world as them-against-us, organic versus conventional, big organic versus small organic, etc. There are some truly major issues coming shortly—economic, agricultural, energy, political—and we need the expertise of many people to develop different perspectives and different solutions. We can learn a lot from each other, but when we view the world from only a black-and-white perspective, we lose many opportunities to learn and to improve." For more information, see the company website at www.lakevieworganicgrain.com.

CHAPTER 6

Which Came First: The Chicken or the Egg?

Which came first, the chicken or the egg?

We won't be able to solve the philosophical puzzle in this chapter, but we can point out that both chickens and their eggs are important food sources in the United States. In fact, more than fifty billion chickens are reared annually as a source of food, for both their meat and their eggs. To clarify the terminology, chickens farmed for meat are called broiler chickens, while those raised for their eggs are referred to as egg-laying hens.

And as for eggs, for a mere seventy calories per egg, they offer complete protein as well as vitamins A, C, and B12, calcium, iron, riboflavin, and phosphorus. Production is increasing every year. In 2009, US egg production was 90.5 billion eggs ($6.17 billion worth), and a year later, in 2010, production was 91.4 billion ($6.52 billion), according to the US Poultry and Egg Association.[64]

In order to qualify as USDA-certified organic, all chickens (egg layers and broilers alike) must be fed only organic feed; they cannot consume any antibiotics (except in case of illness), artificial hormones, or pesticides; and they must have access to the outdoors. For some reason, laying hens, which are smaller, get more space than broilers. But all are required to have room to do their normal chicken foraging in the great outdoors.

An organic egg comes from a laying hen that eats only organic food, receives no growth hormones or antibiotics to boost production, and has access to the outdoors. In rough outlines, the requirements are the same for all organic chickens, whether they are broilers or laying hens.

Playing Chicken with the Ingredients

Much like with their bovine-raising counterparts, most conventional chicken farmers mix a variety of ingredients into their feed to encourage growth and to prevent disease (that is, prophylactically). According to a 2005 report by the Environmental Defense Fund, broiler chickens receive 44 percent of the 26.5 million pounds of antibiotics estimated to be used in the United States each year as feed additives.[65] But don't think that conventionally bred, laying chickens are off the hook, though. They get low-level antibiotics, too. Studies show that chickens that are fed antibiotics often produce eggs with residues of these drugs. According to a study in the *Journal of Agricultural and Food Chemistry* (2000), antibiotics used in chicken feed can linger in a chicken's eggs for up to seven days.

Receiving low-level antibiotics (as we saw in chapter 3: "Where's the Beef?" page 35) can lead to the rise of antibiotic-resistant bacteria. Studies have demonstrated that this is an issue in the chicken industry, much the way it is with beef. A 2011 study by Amy R. Sapkota, PhD, and colleagues in the *Journal of Environmental Health Perspectives* compared conventional poultry farms with those that had recently gone organic. The researchers measured the changes in levels of *entercocci* bacteria and their resistance to seventeen types of antibiotic drugs. The researchers found significantly lower amounts of antibiotic-resistant bacteria (eight distinct types) in organic chicken farms than in conventional chicken farms. "We were surprised to see such dramatic differences in the levels of antibiotic-resistant bacteria in the very first flock at these organic farms," Sapkota said. For instance, Sapkota and colleagues found that fully 67 percent of the *enterococcus* bacterium from conventional poultry farms were resistant to erythromycin, a very common antibiotic; on organic farms, only 18 percent of the bacterium had built up a resistance to this drug.

Not only are antibiotics widespread in commercial meats and poultry, but they affect us humans as well. In a 2001 study published in the *New England Journal of Medicine,* researchers had a dozen volunteers eat resistant strains of *E. faecium* obtained from raw chicken and pork. The researchers, led by Thomas Lund Sorensen, MD, found that these bacteria were present in the volunteers' stool samples for up to two weeks.[66]

Along with their not-medically-indicated antibiotics, an estimated 70 percent of conventionally bred broilers receive Roxarson, a form of arsenic, according to another study that Sapkota and colleagues published in 2006 in the *Applied and Environmental Microbiology Journal.*[67] Roxarson is a chemical intended to improve the growth and feed efficiency in broiler chickens and, sometimes, to improve their pigmentation. It is considered a carcinogen. Organic chickens—and their eggs—do not receive unnecessary antibiotics, nor are they fed arsenic. While the USDA maintains that the levels of these ingredients are too small to have an effect on humans, we may we want to avoid conventionally grown chicken.

Organic Eggs Offer More Vitamins

Organic eggs offer more than just an absence of pesticides and arsenic. Studies show that eating organic eggs is healthier than using conventionally grown eggs. Researchers at Pennsylvania State University's College of Agricultural Science, for instance, found that hens who forage for their food, rather than being fed grain, offer much more nutritious eggs. "Compared to eggs of the commercial hens, eggs from pastured hens had twice as much vitamin E and long-chain omega-3 fats, more than double the total omega-3 fatty acids, and less than half the ratio of omega-6 to omega-3 fatty acids," said Heather Karsten, PhD, lead investigator on the study. To clarify, eggs that are high in omega-6 fatty acids often result in plaque in the arteries—not a good thing, according to Niva Shapira, PhD, Tel Aviv University. "Vitamin A concentration was 38 percent higher in the pastured hens' eggs than in the commercial hens' eggs," Karsten says, "but total vitamin A per egg did not differ."[68]

Why do organic eggs have more nutrients than conventionally grown ones? Perhaps it has to do with what the chickens eat, Karsten suggests. Foraging is what chickens do naturally—and it's better for them than the steady supply of grain that most conventionally tended chickens receive. "Leafy plants like grasses, white clover, red clover, alfalfa, and legumes contain more vitamins and unsaturated fatty acids than standard mash does," says Karsten. In other words, what goes into the chicken comes out in the egg. As Paul Patterson, PhD, professor of poultry science at the university and coinvestigator on the project, explains, "Egg-nutrient levels are responsive to dietary change." The study was published in *Renewable Agriculture and Food Systems* in January 2010.

In addition, research in *Mother Earth News*, published in 2007 and based on USDA data, suggests that there are even more advantages to eggs from hens raised on pasture rather than grain. These include: a third less cholesterol, a quarter less of saturated fat, and seven times as much beta carotene as conventionally grown eggs. These data are similar to what *Mother Earth News* found when it conducted a similar study in 2005.

The History of Chicken in the American Diet

The chicken has a long and noble history in the Western diet. Chickens were first domesticated in Asia, about eight thousand years ago. Well traveled, they came to the United States by way of Europe in the 1400s. They've become pretty popular; these days, the average American eats about eighty pounds of chicken a year, making it our top source of animal protein, according to Local Harvest, an organic and local foods information resource.[69]

Until the early 1900s, chickens were fed some grain and got the rest of their nutrition by foraging. Birds produced eggs for a number of years, then were harvested for food. The early twentieth century's emphasis on specialization and efficiency, though, changed things. By the 1950s and 1960s, egg production became a primary business, and small-scale egg farming all but disappeared, according to Pennsylvania State University's College of Agricultural Science.

The relatively recent emphasis on organic eggs, stemming to about the 1980s or so, has really revived an earlier practice; organic eggs aren't actually anything new. But they are harder to define these days. There seems to be some controversy about what constitutes an "organic egg." The USDA has laid out the basics: no pesticides, synthetic fertilizers, antibiotics, or other prohibited substances. Chickens must be free to roam and have access to the outdoors. But precisely how these last two options work is open for interpretation.

As the Organic Trade Association (OTA) explains, organic egg growers often have different working definition of the details of the USDA standards. Basically, there are three models of organic egg farms, according to the *Cornucopia Institute 2010 Organic Egg Report*:

1. Pasture-based, where birds have mobile housing or permanent housing, with rotated paddocks; this is common on family farms.
2. Permanent housing, where birds have access to the outdoors to some degree, varying from token to adequate; also common on family farms.
3. Industrial-scale organic farms, which often offer "mock" outdoor space or no outdoor access at all.[70]

In essence, then, there are two issues: the health of you and your family, and the conditions under which the hens live. These two issues don't necessarily go hand in hand. When you think about where to put your dollars, you have to decide whether to focus only on your family's health and well-being, or also on that of the chicken.

Talking Chicken

A USDA-certified organic egg is one that was produced with no pesticides, herbicides, synthetic hormones, or fertilizers. These laying chickens cannot be raised in cages and must have access to the outdoors. They can only receive antibiotics in case of infection, not as a preventative or to boost weight gain. Best of all, the USDA regulates this label, so you basically know what you're getting.

Farmers try to promote their products using other terms, which are not regulated by the USDA. That doesn't mean they're untrue, only that you have to take the farmers' word on it. These terms include:

- Free-range or free-roaming: The chickens can wander freely outdoors and eat whatever they want. It typically means they have access to grass, weeds, and insects—not just a square of concrete in the sun. But it's hard to know exactly how much outdoor access the birds get—and how nice their outdoor accommodations are.
- Cage-free: Chickens are allowed to freely roam a building, room, or enclosed area with unlimited access to food and fresh water during their production cycle. This is generally a good thing, as cages are associated with fecal dust and disease-carrying rodents and insects, according to Rodale Press.
- Vegetarian: The chickens were fed a diet free from meat or fish or their byproducts. That means they don't peck any grubs or worms, either.
- Natural: Kind of vague, this term means that the eggs weren't produced by artificial means, so there are no plastic Easter eggs there.
- Humane: This label means that the farmers were nice to their hens.
- Pastured: As we saw above, chickens raised on a pasture produce eggs with more vitamin E and omega fatty acids than grain-fed birds. But, remember, there's no agency or organization regulating this claim.

- Pasteurized: These eggs have been put in a certain amount of heat for a set period of time. Unless labeled as "raw," all eggs sold in the United States have been pasteurized.

An Organic Chicken—or Egg—in Every Pot

People are more and more interested in organic poultry. According to the Organic Trade Association (OTA), poultry represents 62 percent of all sales of organic food. The organization notes that 2011 sales were $33.1 million, a 12.5 percent increase from the previous year.

But there is quite a price difference between organic and standard eggs. It's more expensive to raise organic poultry than conventional poultry because organic feed is more expensive, organic chickens need more space both indoors and outside, and most organic farmers try to treat any illnesses by using antibiotics as little as possible, which is more complicated and expensive than using the drug. Not surprisingly, these costs appear on the price tags for consumers. The United Egg Producers, a nonprofit cooperative of US egg farmers, states that, in 2006, conventional eggs cost about $2.10 a dozen, retail cage-free eggs cost $2.29 a dozen, and organic eggs ran about $3.18 a dozen. But, even so, Americans spent $276 million on organic eggs in 2011, according to the Organic Trade Association.

The Lazy 69 Ranch Story

Year Founded: 1989

  Products: Organic eggs, grass-fed beef

  Where to Buy: Multiple locations in Northern California

Located in Northern California, where the Sierras meet the Cascade Range, the Lazy 69 Ranch is a family ranch that has been raising cattle since 1908. Pam and Henry are the current generation, the fourth to work this land, and they've been at it since 1989. Over the generations, the ranch has grown from twenty-one head of cattle to more than four hundred and fifty head, and encompassing more than 60,000 acres of land.

The ranch also raises free-range chickens, which are fed certified organic feed to supplement what they graze in the pasture, where they spend every day, year round. They live in single hen houses with 3 square feet per bird, as well as 2,000 square feet per bird of outside space. The hens lay eggs for three and a half years, and older birds are taken to a local, free-range animal refuge. The pastured eggs vary in size and color, based on what the birds had been grazing on recently. Bulk sales are also available.

The website attests that "We take an organic, environmentally responsible approach to raising natural, grass-fed beef without the use of hormones, antibiotics or additives." For more information, see the company website at www.lazy69ranch.com .

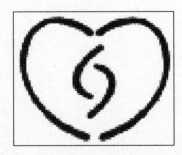

The Neversink Farm Story

Year Founded: 2009

Products: Vegetables, fruits, flowers, honey, eggs, and pork.

Where to Buy: Farmers' markets, retail locations, and upstate New York.

Located in the foothills of New York's Catskill Mountains on the floor of the Neversink Valley, the Neversink Farm sits on twenty acres of mixed woods and pasture. The single-family farm raises vegetables, fruits, honey, eggs, and pork. This wide variety helps to build the circle of sustainability on a small farm.

The hens are heritage breeds. They spend every day from early spring to late fall in the pasture; in the winter, they run around in the snow. The hens also eat organic fruits and vegetables, as well as local, certified organic, whole and ground grains; they never eat animal byproducts.

The farm has more than one hundred types of fruits and vegetables, and a large selection of organic flowers are grown using seeds from farmers' cooperatives and without use of herbicides, pesticides, or fungicides. The bees are kept naturally, using essential oils and organic foods. A community-supported-agriculture-farm membership program (CSA) is available.

The website clarifies the farm's commitment to organic growing: "We follow strict organic growing practices throughout the farm. Organic farming is not just about avoiding petroleum-based fertilizers or pesticides, but about completely removing synthetics and genetically modified organisms from your food." For more information, see the company website at www.neversink-farm.com.

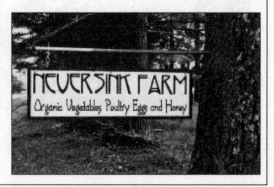

The Bee Heaven Farm Story

Year Founded: 1995

Products: Avocados, honey, eggs, and bananas.

Where to Buy: Local farmers' markets and mail order.

Situated on a five-acre site in Southeast Florida's historic Redland district, just north of Homestead, Bee Heaven Farm started producing avocados in 1999–2000. Then, the single-family farm added organic honey, bananas, and eggs.

The hens eat soy-free, certified-organic feed and harvest gleanings from the farm. They live in single hen houses with 2.5 square feet per bird, as well as 1,500 square feet per bird of outside space. A community supported agriculture program (CSA) farm membership is available.

The company website proclaims: "Our farm has been certified organic since 1997. Our first laying flock began producing in November 2004. Every year, we add some new chicks and cull our roosters and older hens. Our assortment of heritage breeds ensures that every pack of our eggs includes a rainbow of brown, white, green, blue, and speckled eggs, in nearly every size imaginable (we eat the really teeny ones, and the occasional ones that are so big they'd get crushed in the egg carton)." For more information, see the company website at www.pikarco.com.

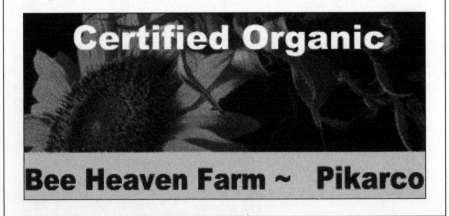

CHAPTER 7

Avoiding GMOs

Genetically modified organisms (GMOs) have permeated our homes, our supermarkets, our fast-food joints, and our fine restaurants. Trying to avoid them is an important task, but it is practically a full-time job these days. This chapter will outline some ways you can lower your risk of consuming GMOs—and the risk of feeding them to your children.

1. Sniff out the most likely GMO culprits.

Certain foods are more likely to be GMO than not. So be particularly careful when considering whether to buy or eat these items: soy products or soybeans, corn, canola, cottonseed, and sugar beets. Let's take a look at each of these foods to see how they are affected by GMOs.

Soybeans: Soybean plants are genetically modified when a gene is taken from bacteria (*Agrobacterium sp.* strain CP4) and inserted into the soybean plant. This makes the plants more resistant to herbicides. The USDA says that 91 percent of soybeans grown in the United States are genetically modified. There are lots of products made from soybeans, including soy flour, soy isolates, soy lecithin, and soy protein. Also, be careful with soy-based products such as tofu, soy milk, and edamame. Most breads contain soy (in the form of lecithin or other dough conditioners). Fresh fruits and vegetables are sometimes sprayed with a waxy coating made of soy. When it comes to processed foods, including luncheon meats, keep an eye out for these terms, which are often code for GMO soy: natural flavor, vegetable oil, and vegetable broth. Oh— and the aspartame in your Diet Coke is made using a fermentation process that involves GMO soy and corn. But the pervasiveness of GMO soybeans doesn't mean there are no organic soybean foods available; just keep reading those labels.

Corn: About 73 percent of US corn is genetically modified. There are three basic varieties of GMO corn. Two types have been genetically modified to kill the insects that eat them, and the third variety was designed to tolerate Monsanto's Roundup herbicide. GMO corn is typically present in high-fructose corn syrup, an ingredient in many processed foods, such as corn flakes and corn chips. Also watch out for corn starch, corn oil, and corn syrup. In addition, GMO corn is often fed to cattle and other livestock, so when you eat beef, pork, or poultry, you may be a secondhand consumer of GMO corn. So, think about opting for grass-fed or free-range livestock. Michael Pollan put it well in his 2006 book, *Omnivore's Dilemma*:

> Corn is in the coffee whitener and Cheez Whiz, the frozen yogurt and TV dinner, the canned fruit and ketchup and candies, the soups and snacks and cake mixes, the frosting and gravy and frozen waffles, the syrups and hot sauces, the mayonnaise and mustard, the hot dogs and bologna, the margarine and shortening, the salad dressings, and the relishes, and even the vitamins.

Canola and Cottonseed: Both of these food items have been modified to resist pests and are fairly prevalent in our food. About 87 percent of cotton (which is made into cottonseed) is GMO, and roughly 75 percent of canola is GMO. Cotton seeds are pressed into cottonseed oil, which is a common ingredient in vegetable oil and margarine; to play it safe, opt for extra virgin olive oil instead.

Sugar Beets: A new concern, GMO sugar beets are becoming more common. According to the USDA, only about 60 percent of sugar beets were GMO in 2008–2009, but the following year, GMO varieties accounted for about 95 percent of sugar beets. And food processors are finding that it's cheaper to get their refined sugar from sugar beets than from cane sugar, so sugar beets are becoming more common. So, if an ingredient is listed as "sugar," not "pure cane sugar," it's a good bet there's some sugar beet in there. Again, check those labels and remember: if it's not marked as "organic," it isn't.

2. Keep an eye on these additional products:

Artificial Sweeteners: Be careful, especially, of aspartame (also known as NutraSweet and Equal or "the little pink or blue packets"), which is created in part by genetically modified microorganisms. And with today's emphasis on weight loss, these sweeteners appear in more than six thousand products, including soft drinks, gum, candy, desserts and mixes, yogurt, tabletop sweeteners, and even some vitamins and sugar-free cough drops.

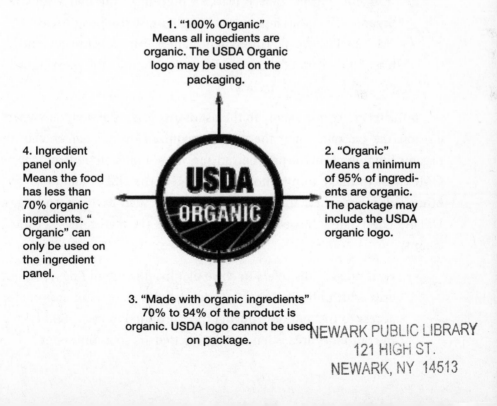

1. "100% Organic"
Means all ingedients are organic. The USDA Organic logo may be used on the packaging.

4. Ingredient panel only Means the food has less than 70% organic ingredients. " Organic" can only be used on the ingredient panel.

2. "Organic"
Means a minimum of 95% of ingredients are organic. The package may include the USDA organic logo.

3. "Made with organic ingredients"
70% to 94% of the product is organic. USDA logo cannot be used on package.

Some Other Vegetables: Certain vegetables are commonly GMO (unless labeled otherwise). These include Hawaiian papaya, zucchini, and yellow squash. Always check the labels.

And more: Also, keep an eye out for honey and bee pollen, which may have been gathered from GMO plants.

3. Learn the terms.

Reading the labels isn't always as easy as it sounds. Labeling isn't always as clear as you'd like. Just remember that the USDA organic seal shows that the product is certified organic and has at least 95 percent organic content. For products with multiple ingredients, such as bread or soup, a USDA organic seal means that each of the ingredients listed has been certified as organic.

Basically, there are three types of organic labels:

1. When a label says "100% organic," it means all ingredients are organic.
2. "Organic" means that at least 95 percent of the ingredients are organic. The other 5 percent, though, must also be non-GMO.
3. "Made with organic (ingredient name)." This label means that at least 70 percent of the ingredients are organic; the remaining 30 percent must be non-GMO.

If the term organic is only in the list of ingredients and not anywhere else on the package, then there is no required overall percentage for organic ingredients in the product, and any nonorganic ingredient may be GMO. Just to make things more complicated, the USDA allows several other voluntary labels for livestock products, such as meat and eggs. USDA's Food Safety Inspection Service verifies the truthfulness of these claims:

• Free-range: This refers to cows that lived in a building, room, or area with unlimited access to food, fresh water, and continuous access to the outdoors during their production cycle. Sometimes the outdoors area is fenced-in or netted-in, sometimes not.

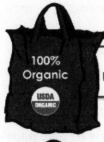

100% Organic
Use of the USDA Organic Seal is optional.

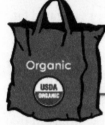

Organic
(95% or more Organic Ingredients)
Use of the USDA Organic Seal is optional.

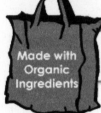

Made with Organic Ingredients
(At least 70% Organic Ingredients)

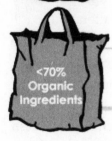

Less than 70% Organic Ingredients
(Organic Ingredients denoted in
ingredient list only)

- Cage-free: Here, cows were allowed to freely roam a building, room, or enclosed area with unlimited access to food and fresh water during their production cycle.
- Natural: Beef, poultry, and egg products labeled as "natural" must be "minimally" processed and cannot contain artificial ingredi-

ents. But this label doesn't say anything about farm practices, only about the processing of the meat or eggs.

- Lean or extra-lean: These terms, as defined by the USDA, specify how much fat is in each gram of beef. Specifically, "lean" means 100 grams (3.5 ounces) of beef must have fewer than 10 grams of fat, 4.5 grams or less of saturated fat, and fewer than 95 milligrams of cholesterol. "Extra lean" means that 100 grams of beef must have fewer than 5 grams of fat, fewer than 2 grams of saturated fat, and fewer than 95 milligrams of cholesterol.
- Hormone-free: There is no certification for this category, though beef labeled "organic" or "grass-fed" must be hormone-free, as certified by the USDA. But if it is just labeled "hormone-free" (and lacks the USDA organic seal), there's no way to know what's in the food.

If that wasn't confusing enough, there are also some labels that don't really provide any information beyond, perhaps, good intentions. Don't be fooled by them. They include:

- Pasture-raised: There's no USDA definition here; the meat industry can use it as it wishes, without government regulation.
- Natural: According to the USDA, a natural product contains "no artificial ingredient or added color and is only minimally processed." Processing cannot fundamentally change the product, and the label must include a specific explanation such as "no artificial ingredients; minimally processed." Incidentally, all fresh meat qualifies as natural; the term says nothing about open space, food (organic or otherwise), or added hormones or antibiotics.
- Humane: Again, this is an unregulated label.
- No added hormones: Federal regulations have never permitted hormones or steroids in poultry, pork, or goat, so this label simply means the producer followed the basic USDA regulations for sale in the United States.

In short: stick with grass-fed beef, though organic would also be fine.

Egg packaging also has its own language. Here are the most common terms:

- Cage-free: This term means that the hens don't live in cages. But that doesn't mean that they have the run of the yard. The American Humane Certified label identifies some, but not all, cage-free eggs.
- Free-range: The USDA certifies that the poultry has been "allowed access to the outside," but does not specify the quality or size of the outside area, nor how much time a given hen gets out there in the open.

4. Decipher the codes on fruits and vegetables.

Those little stickers on fruits and vegetables actually have a purpose, besides making it hard to wash the foods carefully. They are called price look-up (PLU) codes, and they contain numbers that cashiers use to ring you up at the register. These codes aren't mandatory, but they're pretty common, because it makes it easier at the check-out counter. In addition to pricing information, though, these codes provide important information about the product you are buying, at least within the United States. You just need to know what those little numbers mean. According to consumer reports, the first step is to count the number of digits in the code. Then you look at the first digit in the code. Here's a cheat sheet:

- If there are five digits in the code and the first one is a 9, then the item is organic. For instance, small, organic lemons are coded 94033.
- If there are five digits in the code starting with an 8, the item is GMO.
- If there are four digits, starting with a 3 or 4, the product is probably conventionally grown. Small, "regular" lemons, for example, are labeled 4033.

5. Buy whole foods.

Try to use mostly foods that you cook and prepare yourself. Avoid anything that comes in a box or a bag. If you've cooked it, you probably know what's in it. (We hope.) And when you're cooking, think about how you cook. Make sure you're using a GMO-free cooking oil. Soy, cottonseed, canola, butter, and corn oils often contain genetically modified organisms, unless they're labeled as organic. Extra virgin olive oil is probably safest, but—again—read the label.

6. Shop locally.

Most GMO food comes from large, industrial farms, so smaller, local farmers might provide safer food. And there are plenty to choose from; according to Local Harvest, a nonprofit organization devoted to encouraging people to buy locally, there are almost two million farms in the United States, most of them small and family owned. Of course, there's no clear definition of "local"; in densely populated areas, it's pretty nearby, while rural people are often willing to travel a little farther to reach a "local farm." Also, remember that imported produce often contains more pesticides than domestically grown. If you can't find produce within the county, at least stick to the US borders.

Shopping locally may also allow you to speak to the farmer and find out how the farm operates, and whether it uses GMOs. (And maybe even encourage a change in their approach...) Studies show that more than half of the people (about 58 percent) who shop locally do so because they like to know where their food comes from. People also figure they're getting improved quality and freshness of the food items (82 percent) and providing support for the local economy (75 percent).

Local food markets are a growing phenomenon. There are more farmers' markets than ever before. The number of farmers' markets hit 5,274 in 2009, up from 2,756 in 1998, according to the USDA. Sales are up, too. In fact, direct-to-consumer marketing represented about $1.2 billion in current dollar sales in 2007, according to the 2007 Census of Agriculture, compared with $551 million a decade earlier.

7. Grow your own food.

If you grow it, you know whether you used organic or GMO seeds, you know what fertilizer did—or did not—go on your plants. And you'd probably know if you sprayed the plant with an herbicide or pesticide. If you have more space, say a side or backyard, you can plant vegetables in seasonal rotation; there's nothing like picking a tomato, then going inside to cut it up for a very fresh salad. It's probably more of a challenge for city folks. If you only have a little space for "farming," use a planter on the windowsill or balcony to grow herbs and fruit trees.

Children often like growing food, too. Even preschoolers can become quite proficient at knowing which vegetables to pick. Some easy-to-grow plants are radishes, herbs, and peas, and once you experience success, you might find you want to branch out to other beloved fruits and veggies. Most important, children who grow their own vegetables often have a good understanding about the connections between soil, food, and their own health. Role modeling is always the best way to teach. And if a child grew the veggies, he or she might be more apt to eat them when they appear on the dinner plate.

8. Be careful when dining out.

Start by picking restaurants that cook meals from scratch and don't use packaged, processed mixes and sauces; these are more likely to have GMO ingredients. Fast-food and chain restaurants are more likely to be problematic than mom-and-pop places.

Don't be afraid to ask questions, especially if it's a restaurant you go to regularly. If there's a knowledgeable server or chef, that person can guide you through the menu to help you avoid GMO foods. Ask about what type of cooking oil they use at the restaurant. Usually, when someone tells you they use vegetable oil or butter, they're talking about soy, cottonseed, canola, or corn oil. These are often GMO—unless they are certified organic. Olive oil is probably safest, but be careful that it's not a blend; some restaurants mix canola and olive oils.

The good news is that once you've been through a menu, you probably won't need to ask a second time. Chances are the restaurant won't suddenly switch from organic to GMO—especially if they know the customers are watching. And you told them that! Also, by showing the restaurant that you care about what is in the foods you order and eat, the owner or chef might be more likely to try to avoid genetically modified ingredients in the future.

CHAPTER 8

Detoxification: Nutritional and Dietary Approaches

W e humans sit at the top of the food chain. So we ingest, along with the vitamins and nutrients, everything that everyone else has eaten along the way. If farmers use pesticides and herbicides to help grow the grain that livestock consumes, then, well, some of that ends up in our systems as well. And exposure to these sorts of toxins builds up over time, a process that is called *bioaccumulation*.

As we have seen in the earlier chapters, genetically modified organisms are only one of many concerning substances that are imposed on our bodies. Within food alone, as we have seen, we often unwittingly ingest synthetic hormones, herbicides, pesticides, and unnecessary antibiotics. While we can work to eliminate these items from our diets (see chapter 7: "Avoiding GMOs," page 97), that doesn't help the fact that we've been taking those chemicals into our bodies for years. The Southwest College of Naturopathic Medicine and Health Sciences notes that, according to the CDC, more than 80 percent of all illnesses have environmental and lifestyle causes. And, according to the CDC's Agency for Toxic Substances and Disease Registry, at least two-thirds of all cancers in the United States are caused by environmental factors.

Many people choose to cleanse their bodies of these toxins, a process often called "detoxification." Detoxification technically means simply getting rid of toxins or poisons. The process is nothing new; Native Americans used sweat lodges and Indians used Panchakarma. At one point, the term referred primarily to overcoming addiction or achieving weight loss. But over the years, the term has come to include cleansing the body of the chemicals that are in our food and environment. One of the most popular approaches in alternative medicine, detoxification is based on the principle that illness is, at least in part, caused by the build-up of toxins in your system.

Detoxification is one of the best ways to recover your health, according to the Southwest College of Naturopathic Medicine and Health Sciences. (Naturopathic medicine works with nature to restore people's health, according to the American Association of Naturopathic Physicians.) Typically, according to the College, the first step is to get rid of exposure to all toxic or allergenic substances. This includes heavy metals, chemicals, radiation (from x-rays, power lines, cell phones, computer screens, and microwaves), smog, polluted water, foods, drugs, caffeine, alcohol, perfume, excess noise, and stress. Not the easiest thing to do in the twenty-first century.

There's no standard practice in the field of detoxification, according to a study by Jason Allen, ND, and colleagues, published in the *Journal of Alternative and Complementary Medicine* in 2011.[71] Rather, there are many types of alternative therapies available, too many to list here. But we will try to lay out the basic therapies and provide enough information for you to decide whether you'd like to look into them further. Remember— you may have to experiment and figure out what approach or approaches work best for you.

Nutritional and Dietary Detox

First of all, there is no such thing as a detox diet, says Gary Null, PhD, who is considered one of the top natural healing gurus in the United States. He explains that when we think about cleansing our bodies, we should remember that every single morsel we eat and every single drop of liquid we drink has an effect on our bodies. Not immediately, of course, but cumulatively. No one gets lung cancer from one cigarette, no one gets cirrhosis of the liver from a single sip of vodka, Null points out. Just because there's no immediate, observable response to a toxin doesn't mean the body hasn't been affected.

The notion of moderation in all things doesn't work for the human body. "How do you figure out what a moderate amount of cadmium is?" asks Null, who is also a journalist, author, and talk show host. There is no standard, only average; averages are not a true reflection of society. When we talk about the average amount of meat an American eats, the "average" includes vegetarians; when we talk about the average amount of sugar intake, we are including diabetics, who pretty much avoid consuming sugar altogether.

The liver works continually to detoxify the body, but it can only do so much. Eventually, the body reaches a tipping point, and a symptom appears: an inflamed joint, a clogged artery. When the body manifests symptoms, it is not the beginning of a health concern—it is a sign that things have gone too far. And the typical American diet, full of GMOs, really tests those limits.

One approach to cleansing out the GMOs and other harmful substances is detoxification. It can take one to three years to get all the residual effects out of the body. Anyone planning to detoxify his or her body will need a health-care practitioner to oversee and monitor the process, though the practitioner may refer patients to other experts for particular processes, such as acupuncture. There are a variety of approaches to detoxification, which we discuss in this chapter; they are all complementary, none are contradictory, asserts Null. The entire time, your health-care provider should monitor you for cancer markers, immune modality markers, and other issues.

Vitamin C Drip

Vitamin C is one of the most widely sold vitamins; in 2007, there was more vitamin C sold in the United States than any other vitamin, amounting to roughly $884 million dollars. While it is helpful to take a tablet or two, an intravenous (IV) vitamin C drip has particular medical benefits and is a very common treatment among complementary and alternative (CAM) health practitioners.

A survey by Sebastian J. Padayatty, MD, and colleagues of the National Institutes of Health in 2010 found that the vast majority of CAM practitioners frequently administered IV vitamin C, mostly to treat infection (44 percent), cancer (19 percent), or other conditions, including fatigue (37 percent). Patients received, on average, 28 grams every four days, with twenty-two total treatments per patient. Total dosing vials of IV vitamin C sold in the United States were approximately 750,000 in 2006 and 855,000 in 2008. When patients were screened properly, there were "surprisingly few" side effects.[72]

Not only is this a popular treatment, but studies show that it is effective. In 2005, a National Institutes of Health (NIH) researcher, Qui Chen, found that vitamin C, in pharmacologic concentrations, killed cancer cells while leaving healthy cells alone.[73] Similarly, a 2009 study in China found that rats given intravenous, high-dose vitamin C showed improvement in tumor volume and tumor growth.[74]

The treatment has been found to be especially helpful for cancer patients, when administered side by side with conventional Western treatments. In 2007, a Korean study of terminal cancer patients showed that an IV vitamin C drip improved their quality of life. Patients received 10 grams of IV vitamin C twice a day for three days, followed by a 4 gram vitamin C pill for a week. Patients reported that they felt much better, physically, emotionally, and cognitively. They also reported feeling significantly less tired and experiencing less nausea, vomiting, and appetite loss.

Again, the treatment was found to be safe and effective. Similar results were found in a 2011 study of breast cancer patients in Germany.[75]

Chelation Therapy

When heavy metals need to be removed, this is an effective technique. Patients have an intravenous drip of ethylenediaminetetraacetic acid (EDTA) over a period of five to thirty sessions. This medication seeks out and binds to minerals in your bloodstream, creating a compound that leaves your body in your urine, according to the Mayo Clinic.

Chelation has been scientifically proven to rid the body of excess or toxic metals, notes the National Institutes of Health, and it has been approved by the FDA to treat lead poisoning and toxicity from other heavy metals. The NIH has conducted preliminary tests of chelation therapy as a treatment for coronary disease, and it has been found to be of some benefit. Preliminary results of the study were presented in November 2012, though final conclusions are still pending.[76]

It is an increasingly popular course of treatment, too, according to the National Heart Lung and Blood Institute of the National Institutes of Health. Between 2002 and 2007, use of chelation therapy grew by nearly 68 percent, reaching a high of 111,000 people.

Juicing

Every American should eat between five and thirteen servings of fruits and vegetables a day, according to the Harvard School of Public Health. Most people don't even come close; if you don't count potatoes—and most nutritionists consider them a starch rather than a vegetable—most Americans consume just three servings of fruits and vegetables a day, notes Harvard.

Juicing offers an alternative, hopefully, a tasty and efficient one. Advocates suggest you can drink more vegetables than you eat—and juicing allows the body to absorb the vitamins and antioxidants more easily, according to PBS. And some point out that juicing allows you to vary your veggies more than you might otherwise.

Some people get their juice at a juice bar or health food store, but if you do that, make sure to read the labels so you don't pour something down your throat that you wouldn't want in your body. You can also get your own juicer and do it yourself; that way, you know exactly what's in each sip. Of course, it's best to go with organic fruits and vegetables (see chapter 4: "The Dirty Dozen"). And don't prep for the week by making a bucketful of juice on Sunday night—these juices won't keep more than a day or two.

Start with celery, fennel (anise), and cucumbers, suggests author Joseph Mercola, DO, as these are the easiest to digest and tolerate, even though they aren't the most nutrient-dense. When you're ready, Mercola recommends stepping up to red and green leaf lettuce, romaine lettuce, endive, escarole, and spinach. Pros may want to add cabbage, Chinese cabbage, and bok choy. Some people add herbs such as parsley and cilantro. And for the pièce de résistance, add a leaf or two of one of these relatively bitter greens for extra nutrient kick: kale, collard greens, dandelion greens, and mustard greens. To add a little zest to your drink, Mercola suggests adding lemons, limes, cranberries, or fresh ginger.

There's plenty of research indicating the importance of fruits and vegetables. Some studies have found that it is useful in delaying the onset of Alzheimer's Disease[76] or general cognitive decline;[78] one study emphasizes the importance of cruciferous vegetables, such as broccoli and cabbage, legumes, and green leafy vegetables. Several other studies have found that regular fruit and vegetable intake can add to heart health.[79] Another study showed that fruits and vegetables can decrease chances of contracting cataracts.[79]

A study performed in 2007 found that not only are fruits and vegetables helpful, but it pinpointed an amount.[80] By conducting a meta-analysis of prospective cohort studies, the researchers at the Blood Pressure Unit at the University of London found that boosting fruit and vegetable consumption from less than three servings daily to more than five is related to a 17 percent reduction in risk of coronary heart disease. So—juice it up.

Supplements

Often, when someone worries about getting enough of particular vitamins, such as vitamin C during the flu season, that person takes a vitamin pill or supplement. But supplements can also include minerals, fiber, fatty acids, or amino acids—just about anything that might be missing from or insufficient in someone's diet.

This is a very common approach, according to the National Institutes of Health's National Center for Complementary and Alternative Medicine (NCCAM). A national survey conducted in 2007 found that 17.7 percent of American adults had used dietary supplements (other than vitamins and minerals) in the past twelve months. The most popular among adults were: fish oil/omega 3/DHA (37.4 percent); glucosamine (19.9 percent); echinacea (19.8 percent); flaxseed oil or pills (15.9 percent); and ginseng (14.1 percent).

Here is a list of some potentially useful supplements, along with a little information about their uses, courtesy of the University of Maryland Center for Integrative Medicine. Many of them are antioxidants, which protect the body from free radicals. Free radicals damage cells through a process called oxidation, which, over time, can lead to a number of chronic illnesses. Research suggests that getting more antioxidants through diet can protect against free radicals and lower the risk of heart disease and cancer, but it isn't clear whether the same is true of antioxidant supplements. Remember: there is always the possibility of side effects or interactions with any other medications you may be taking, so only use supplements under the guidance of your health-care provider.

Quercetin, a flavonoid, is an antioxidant that may help protect against heart disease and cancer. Researchers suspect that it may also help reduce allergy symptoms, including runny nose, watery eyes, and hives. It is generally considered safe, but you should take periodic breaks when on it.

CO-Q-10 (Coenzyme Q10) is an antioxidant that is found naturally in the body and helps convert food into energy. Researchers believe it can help with heart-related conditions, improve blood pressure, and lower cholesterol. There is also some evidence that it may improve immune function in people with HIV or AIDS, increase male fertility, help prevent migraines, improve exercise ability in people with angina, and help Parkinson's patients. It is generally considered safe. Carnitine (or L-carnitine), another antioxidant, helps convert fat into energy. Some evidence suggests that it can work alongside conventional treatment to stabilize angina and increase sperm count and motility. It is sometimes prescribed for kidney disease. Side effects are generally mild.

Milk thistle (Silybum marianum) has been used as an herbal remedy for thousands of years. It is often recommended as treatment for alcoholic hepatitis, alcoholic cirrhosis, and viral hepatitis. Scientific studies have shown that some of the substances in milk thistle, especially a flavonoid and antioxidant called silymarin, can help protect the liver from toxins such as drugs. Silymarin is thought to have anticancer qualities. It is generally regarded as safe.

Dandelion leaf is a diuretic that is thought to increase the excretion of drugs from the body. But be careful, as it may interact with prescription medications.

Sulfur is a naturally occurring mineral usually found near hot springs and volcanic craters. As a supplement, it comes in two forms: dimethyl sulfoxide (DMSO) and methylsulfonylmethane (MSM). Both can help alleviate pain. MSM is thought to help in joint health and arthritis, though there is little scientific evidence to support this. Researchers believe MSM is safe.

Magnesium aids every organ in the body, especially teeth and bones. It activates enzymes, helps with energy production, and regulates levels of calcium, copper, zinc, potassium, vitamin D, and other nutrients in the body. There is conflicting evidence about whether it aids in asthma, hearing loss, migraine headaches, PMS, and blood pressure. Common side effects include upset stomach and diarrhea. Beta-carotene, an antioxidant, is thought to protect against cancer, but it actually increases the risk for people who smoke or drink heavily. It may also slow the progression of macular degeneration and protect against sun sensitivity (though not sunburn). Side effects can include skin discoloration, loose stools, bruising, and joint pain.

Glucosamine is produced naturally in the body and is vital to building cartilage. While some studies suggest it can help osteoarthritis (OA), it's not certain that it can help repair or grow new cartilage or protect existing cartilage. Researchers think it can, however, reduce OA pain and improve functioning, and reduce joint swelling and stiffness. Considered safe, glucosamine may cause insulin to work less effectively and may raise blood pressure and cholesterol levels.

Other Important Ways to Detox

Complementary and alternative (CAM) approaches to detoxification and other medical concerns are becoming increasingly popular—and increasingly mainstream, according to a 2011 study by the Health Forum, a subsidiary of the American Hospital Association (AHA), and Samueli Institute, a nonprofit organization devoted to studying alternative health modalities. Sometimes CAM is called integrative medicine.

Researchers, led by Sita Ananth, director of knowledge services for Samueli Institute, found that almost half of the hospitals that responded to the survey (about 42 percent) said they offered one or more CAM therapies in 2011, up from 37 percent in 2007. And patient requests are the big reason; the survey found that 85 percent of responding hospitals chose to offer CAM services due to patient demand, and 70 percent said that clinical effectiveness was their top reason. Interestingly, the majority of hospitals that offered CAM were urban hospitals (72 percent).

Nearly two-thirds of hospitals offering alternative services provided massages on an outpatient basis, and half offered pet therapy in the hospital. About 40 percent of these hospitals offered acupuncture or music and art therapies, said the report, based on an American Hospital Association survey conducted in March 2010. One in five alternative-friendly hospitals provides Reiki therapy. Though almost three-quarters of the executives of the hospitals providing unconventional therapies (70 percent) said they were doing so because they were clinically effective, less than half (42 percent) said they use patients' health outcomes to gauge the success of the alternative medicine programs.

Deep-Breathing Exercises

Considered one of the best ways to decrease stress in the body, deep-breathing exercises are often called a "mind-body therapy." This is one of the most popular alternative medical procedures, used by 12.7 percent of Americans, according to the National Center for Complementary and Alternative Medicine (NCCAM) of the National Institutes of Health (NIH). It is also one of the most flexible and portable methods of self-treatment; you can do deep breathing just about any time, anywhere, in most any position, and it usually takes no more than ten minutes.

The process is simple. It often helps to start sitting down, legs uncrossed, and eyes closed. Then, inhale slowly and deeply through your nose; most people count to ten to ensure that they're doing it slowly enough. Then you exhale completely, counting to ten again. You can repeat this process five to ten times, several times a day, according to NCCAM. Some experts say that this technique becomes more effective over the years. It is considered extremely safe.

Meditation

A simple, fast way to reduce stress, meditation helps you focus your attention and suspend all outside thoughts. The goal is to increase calmness, physical relaxation, and a sense of balance. And it is one of the most common alternative medical treatments in the country; the US Centers for Disease Control and Prevention (CDC) estimates that 12.7 percent of the American population used this technique in 2007.

Despite its association with the New Age lifestyle, meditation is nothing new. It has been around for thousands of years. At one point, it was considered a way to connect with sacred and mystical forces. These days, we see it as a way to connect more fully with ourselves. According to the Mayo Clinic, meditation can help you gain a new perspective on a stressful situation, build stress-management skills, increase self-awareness, focus on the present (rather than all those bothersome could-have, should-have thoughts), and reduce negative emotions.

There are several ways to meditate, the clinic explains. You can focus on a mental image that you find relaxing, such as a bucolic outdoor scene; you can repeat a mantra, which is a calming word, thought, or phrase; you can focus on a sense of love and gratitude; or you can concentrate on the immediate experience, such as the feeling of breath in your body or the sensation of your feet on the floor. However you meditate, though, the point is to block out all stressful and unwanted thoughts.

Remember, though, that it is common for your mind to wander every so often, even for the most experienced meditators. If you worry about your lack of focus, you have simply traded one source of anxiety for another. Many people combine deep breathing with meditation. Unless you're in danger of missing your train or subway stop, this is another fairly safe method of alternative therapy.

Acupuncture

Tracing its roots to China, acupuncture has been around for about twenty-five hundred years. It is sometimes used to treat specific aches and pains and sometimes to gain a general feeling of wellness. These days, more and more people are turning to acupuncture to cleanse their body—of genetically modified organisms and other stresses of the twenty-first century. Acupuncturists stimulate specific points on the body by inserting very slender metal needles through the skin, a process that most people say does not hurt. In the United States, acupuncturists must attend a four-year graduate program to be licensed to practice.

The therapy is based on the theories of Chinese traditional medicine, which holds that the body contains two opposing forces—yin and yang. Chinese medicine explains that illness and disease occur when there is an imbalance between the two that blocks the flow of chi (pronounced "chee"), or life force energy. Acupuncture is said to remove these blockages and restore health. There are several styles of acupuncture, and all are believed to be safe, if practiced correctly using sterile needles. Use is on the rise; in the United, States, 4.2 percent of Americans used acupuncture in 2002 (8.19 million people), rising to 6.3 percent in 2007 (14.01 million people), according to a study by Yan Zhang, PhD and colleagues at Texas Tech University. It's not used just in the United States, though; the British National Health Service estimated that four million acupuncture sessions were provided in 2009.

Some studies attest to its effectiveness. According to the World Health Organization, acupuncture is most useful in stopping or lessening pain, protecting the body against infection, and regulating certain physiological functions. Americans tend to come to acupuncture, according to the Texas Tech study, seeking assistance in general wellness (42.3 percent), enhanced energy (24.0 percent), and improved immune function (21.7 percent).

A 2012 study published in the Archives of Internal Medicine looked at almost eighteen thousand patients in the United States, UK, Germany, Spain, and Sweden and found that acupuncture is an effective treatment for chronic pain. Specifically, patients suffering from chronic headaches; back, neck, or shoulder pain or osteoarthritis found acupuncture to be significantly more effective than typical pain treatment.[82]

While researchers don't really know *why* acupuncture works, according to Richard L. Nahin of NIH's National Center for Complementary and Alternative Medicine, studies show that it does. It is considered extremely safe, assuming a qualified practitioner and sterilized needles. But you might not feel the effects immediately; experts advise having several sessions before deciding whether the treatment works for you.

Yoga

One of the oldest forms of medicine, yoga traces its roots back more than five thousand years to India. The practice of yoga encompasses meditation, breathing, and physical postures. In the United States and throughout the Western world, the practice of yoga has come to mean a series of poses or exercises. But originally, the poses and breathing were seen as a way to help practitioners meditate, forcing them to think about something other than daily life and its stresses. Yoga is very popular within the United States, one of the top ten CAM practices, according to NCCAM. In 2007, the NCCAM found that more than 13 million adults and more than 1.5 million children had practiced yoga in the previous year.

Research shows that yoga can lower stress and promote health. One study, by Janice Kiecolt-Glaser, PhD, and colleagues at the Ohio State University of Medicine, found that yoga can minimize the body's response to stress; the researchers suggest that long-term practice could have substantial health benefits. Yoga is generally considered low-impact and safe for healthy people *when practiced appropriately under the guidance of a well-trained instructor.* Some studies have suggested that yoga can reduce heart rate and blood pressure, as well as help relieve anxiety and depression, according to NCCAM.

As with other forms of alternative medical therapy, there are many types of yoga practices. The *Yoga Journal* outlines a number of these, including:

- Ashtanga: A fast-paced series of sequential postures, this system is based on six series of poses that increase in difficulty. Students usually work at their own pace.
- Jivamukti: This practice is highly meditative but physically challenging. Classes emphasize forward bends, backbends, and inversions.
- Iyengar yoga: This type of yoga requires intense focus on each position. Practitioners typically hold these poses longer than in other yogic practices, so they can pay close attention to their precise muscular and skeletal alignment.
- Bikram yoga: This style of yoga takes place in rooms that are close to 100 degrees in temperature. The intention is to sweat the toxins out of the body. If you choose this style, be sure to bring plenty of water.
- Kundalini yoga: A practice that incorporates postures, dynamic breathing techniques, and chanting and meditating on mantras.

Some yoga instructors offer sessions geared to people with particular medical concerns, such as balance issues.

Remember that everyone's body is different, and you should modify the yoga postures to suit your individual abilities. Once you find a style of yoga that you enjoy, be sure to select an instructor who can help you figure out and make these modifications.

Reiki Therapy

Reiki is the Japanese term for universal life energy. In this energy-healing therapy, practitioners place their hands lightly on or hold them just above the patient. The goal, according to NCCAM, is to recharge, realign, and rebalance the human energy fields and facilitate the patient's own healing power. It is based on an Eastern belief in an energy that supports the body's own ability to heal itself.

Studies have found Reiki to be beneficial. A 2010 study by John Gruzelier, PhD, and his students at the University of London found that patients receiving Reiki therapy showed a decrease in the symptoms of illness, even though they started out with higher "scores" on self-reported symptoms and stress. These researchers wanted to rule out any psychological effect of receiving Reiki by giving some patients no-touch Reiki and some no Reiki at all.[83]

An earlier study, published in 2005 in the *Orthopedic Nursing Journal* by Ellen M. DiNucci, MA, at Stanford University, looks at various studies, finding that it helps with wound healing, and has positive effects on pain and anxiety.[84] Similarly, researchers have found that patients report an increased calmness due to Reiki.[85]

And in another study, A. G. Shore, in 2004, followed patients being treated for mild depression and stress and found that Reiki can have long-term effects on depression and stress. Specifically, Shore found that a full year after treatment, patients who received Reiki therapy were still doing better than their untreated counterparts in terms of depression, stress, and hopelessness.[86]

It is a popular therapy that, according to the Center for Reiki Research, has been practiced for nearly a century. More than 1.2 million American adults, approximately half of the US adult population, used an energy-healing therapy such as Reiki in 2006, according to NCCAM. Researchers report that Reiki is safe and has no serious side effects.

Sweat Therapy

Saunas, which are a room or house designed to provide wet or dry heat, have been shown to aid in detoxification because they allow us to sweat out the toxins through our skin. Sessions intended to reduce blood pressure and enhance blood flow and cardiac functioning typically last about fifteen minutes, though sessions for detoxification may be longer—and should be medically monitored, according to a study published by Walter Crinnion, N.D., in *Alternative Therapies in Health and Medicine Journal* in 2007.[87] Many people take a cold shower after using a sauna. Saunas are considered particularly helpful for those with environmentally induced illnesses.

And it's pretty safe; although sitting in a sauna can cause changes in cardiovascular and hormone functioning, most healthy adults and children do just fine in a sauna, according to a study published in the *American Journal of Medicine* by researchers Minna L. Hannuksela, MD, Samer Ellahham, MD, at the University of Oulu in Finland.[88]

Massage Therapy

Massage therapy is one of the most popular types of alternative medical treatment in the country. NCCAM estimates that about eighteen million US adults and seven hundred thousand children received at least one massage in 2006. Most people find massage therapy to be relaxing—and they also feel that it promotes their overall well-being.

The procedure is simple. Patients usually lie on a table in loose-fitting clothing or are covered only with a sheet. Sometimes, the massage therapist uses oil or lotion to reduce friction on the skin. Using their hands, massage therapists manipulate muscle and connective tissue. Sessions tend to be relaxing and can last anywhere from twenty minutes to an hour.

Most massage therapists are licensed professionals, according to the CDC. Most states have licensing requirements for massage therapists. The American Massage Therapy Association (AMTA) notes that there are more than three hundred fifty accredited massage therapy schools and programs throughout the United States.

"Medical massage" is actually a broad term that encompasses a variety of styles, according to the State University of New York. These include Swedish medical massage (which uses five styles of long, flowing strokes); deep tissue massage (which focuses on the muscles below the top, surface muscles); acupressure (where the practitioner applies physical pressure to acupuncture points); and Shiatsu (which uses the same energy meridians as acupressure and incorporates stretching).

At least one study shows that massage works to improve body functioning. Research published by Mark H. Rapaport, MD, and colleagues at Cedars-Sinai Medical Center in the *Journal of Alternative Complementary Medicine* in 2010 finds that a single session of Swedish massage therapy produces measurable, biologic effects on neuroendocrine and immune function.

As you can see, there are many ways to approach cleansing the body from environmental and food toxins. There are methods you can try by yourself, approaches that require an accredited practitioner, and ways that demand ongoing medical monitoring. Try whatever sounds interesting, and pick the modality or modalities that feel right for you and your family.

CHAPTER 9

Future Trends

A mericans are changing the way we look at food. We are starting to see it less as a hobby and something to do with our hands while we watch television or drive our cars, and more of a way to fuel our bodies in a healthy way. We are focusing on sustainability, trying to take better care of the planet and make sure that it will be viable for our children and our children's children (and hopefully beyond that). We want to eat better—better for us, for our families, and for the world.

Without question, the organic food movement is growing worldwide. The question, as Dr. John David Paull explains, is how much momentum it has. As of 2010, some countries have set goals for themselves: France, for instance, would like to be 20 percent organic by 2020. And some countries have already made substantial progress; in Liechtenstein for instance, 29.7 percent of the agricultural land is farmed organically. Other countries have made crop-specific goals: Mexico's coffee production is 30 percent organic, and 70 percent of the Dominican Republic's banana production is organic, as Paull notes.[89] Will that translate into 100 percent organic by the time our kids reach middle age? It's hard to tell.

Paull sets out two separate predictions: The first predicts that organic food production will continue to grow geometrically at 13.2 percent a year, which means we'll reach 100 percent at about 2048. The other scenario assumes organic agriculture continues to grow arithmetically at 22.8 percent a year, which will land us at 100 percent in the far-off year of 1553.

So, which will it be?

This chapter looks at several trends within the world of organic agriculture. First, we consider the challenges that hard economic times have placed on the organic food movement. Specifically, we look at some of the alternatives that are arising to enable moderate-income people to eat organically. Then, we consider the changing demographics of those buying organic; more and more Asian and Latino Americans are heading toward the organic aisles when they shop. We look at the controversial issue of mandatory labeling in the United States; while the measure has been defeated in various states and localities, the issue is far from decided, and we can assume we will be reading headlines about the topic in the years to come. We also talk about the Non-GMO Project, an effort that goes beyond USDA organic certification to promote food that is totally without genetically modified organisms. And, finally, we take a look around the world at the varying approaches that different countries are taking—at least as of this writing—toward the important issue of what we eat.

Budget Organic

We are coming through some rough economic times. Most of us have had to pinch our pennies at least a little bit, and while we are optimistic, we are still careful. As a result, there's been increased interest in various ways of eating healthily on a budget. Some of the ways Americans are achieving this goal is by buying private label organics, and by connecting more strongly with farmers—through farmers' markets, community-supported agriculture, and buying clubs—and by shopping at food co-ops.

As we talked about earlier, more and more people are shopping locally—using many different definitions of "local" food. And they often do so because they want to know more about where their food came from and how it was grown. According to the USDA, sales directly from farmer to consumer are increasing.

As the economy continues to struggle, so do many Americans. But that doesn't mean we don't want to eat healthy food free of genetically modified organisms, pesticides and herbicides, and synthetic hormones. It just means that when we shop for organic food, we keep an eye on our wallets. Private labels and buying clubs are two ways to save money while buying organic.

Private Label Organic. Store brands, products sold under a retail store's private label, have a lot of aliases: they are called private label, private brands, house brands, own brands, and retailer brands, according to the Private Label Manufacturers Association. Chances are, there are some in your kitchen (and bathroom and garage, too). Almost every one (91 percent) buys store brands at least some of the time, according to Consumer Edge Insight. In your home—and in the store—they sit right next to manufacturer brands.

Who makes these private label products? Large manufacturers who make their own products, as well as private label items; smaller manufacturers who focus in private label products; and major retailers and wholesalers who produce private label items for their own stores.

At one time, people were suspicious of private label brands. But no more. Consumer Edge Insight has found that while a good number (31 percent) of consumers think manufacturer brands are better than store brands, almost as many (27 percent) feel that store brands offer comparable quality. According to the Hartman Group, in 2007, 10 percent of shoppers consistently buy private label products when they're shopping for organics, and another 21 percent do so occasionally.[90]

Store brands come in every product line, from office supplies to hardware, and from cleaning products to organic food. And all store brands must meet all federal requirements. So, anything labeled "USDA-Certified Organic" must meet all the USDA standards. It's just as organic as a manufacturer-branded organic food item. And the best part? Store brands cost about a third less than national brands, according to PLMA, thanks to the lower promotional and advertising costs.

For example, Safeway's O Organics brand offers more than 300 certified organic products, including dairy and eggs, fruit and vegetables, snacks and seasonings, and baby formula and toddler food. Other private labels at major department store chains include Kroger's Simple Truth Organic, Whole Foods' 365 Everyday Value, and Lowe's Full Circle. And all come with lower price tags than "regular" organic products.

Farmers' Markets. These communal spaces are a win-win. Farmers from family farms, as well as small- and medium-sized facilities, can offer their products directly to the public. And the mostly urban clientele has access to fresh food, straight from the farm. Farmers, markets are actually nothing new. At one point, they were pretty standard, especially in cities. But then the food system consolidated, and interstate highways (and the trucking industry) were developed in the early- and mid-twentieth century. By 1970, there were only about 340 farmers' markets left in the entire country, according to the Union of Concerned Scientists.

But now farmers' markets are back in vogue. According to the USDA, there were 7,864 farmers' markets registered nationwide as of August 2012, and the numbers are increasing. There were more than 20 farmers' markets in 2011 for each one that existed in 1970, according to the Union for Concerned Scientists. In Vermont, farmers' markets grew 177 percent between 1995 and the year 2010, according to the Northeast Organic Farming Association of Vermont (NOFA-VT). Farmers' markets tend to carry a wide range of seasonal fruits and vegetables as well as dairy products, honey, and some baked goods. Since they include a variety of farmers, there is often plenty of diversity in items for sale. And, chances are, it's all farm-fresh.

Shoppers should be aware that not everything sold at a farmer's market is certified organic. Check the labels, or even just ask the farmer behind the counter. There's usually more organic food here, though, than in traditional shopping outlets. A 2010 NOFA-VT study found that 53 percent of food items at Vermont farmers' markets were organic.

Farmers' markets are usually a good way to save money, notes NOFA-VT. The association's 2010 study of Vermont foods found that every organic food item, except potatoes, cost less at farmers' markets than at co-ops or grocery stores. Specifically, the study found that organic items were 38.8 percent cheaper than the same item at a grocery store, and 28.7 percent less expensive than at a co-op.

Beyond that, since you're talking directly with the farmers themselves, shoppers can always try to bargain prices down. That might work, especially on a slow day, if you're offering to buy in bulk, or at the very end of the day at the market, when farmers are about to load up unsold food and take it home. There's no guarantee that you'll get a deal, but it's worth a shot.

CSA. Community Supported Agriculture (CSA) means that a group of people become "shareholders" of a farm by pledging to pay the anticipated cost of running the farm, including a salary for the farmer. In return, shareholders typically get a bag, box, or carton of food every week during the harvesting season. Some CSAs deliver the farm-fresh food right to your door. Others ask members (or shareholders) to do some work on the farm. At the Quail Hill Farm in New York, for instance, shareholders do almost all the harvesting of crops. Remember, though, that the produce will probably be scarcer at the beginning of the season and by the end, you may have more fruit and vegetables than you know what to do with.

This approach gives the farmers some up-front capital to invest, as well as a level of financial security. It helps consumers because they get lower prices and fresher produce; Quail Hill Farm, for instance, grows twenty types of herbs and more than forty types of fruits and vegetables, plus eggs and honey. And kids who are involved in harvesting, or even just picking up vegetables from "their farm," are more likely to chow down when the veggies hit their dinner plate.

Part of the CSA concept is the notion of shared risk. A drought or hurricane, for instance, would hit shareholders as well as farmers. But think about it this way: even people relying exclusively on supermarkets for their produce will feel the pinch of a poor growing season. Just be aware that you may not be able to rely on a CSA to supply all your produce.

The concept of CSA was developed more than two decades ago, in Japan and Chile. But, according to Rodale Institute, the European community-supported farms were the ones that really influenced the development of CSA in the United States, in the late 1980s. The USDA notes that there were 12,549 CSA farms in the United States in 2007.

Buying Clubs. Buying clubs are a booming business, and they're not as complicated as they sound. Basically, a group of people pools their time, resources, and buying power to save money on quality, healthy foods. They work directly with a distributor, who then ships in bulk quantities—and at wholesale prices. They are similar to CSAs, but it's typically more of a pay-as-you-go plan, rather than a long-term commitment.

Buying clubs often operate out of someone's home or office. Shipments arrive at a delivery location where club members can then sort the products and take home their goodies. In many cases, there's no membership fee or commitment; all you get is low-cost, organic food items. The precise rules, though, vary from buying club to buying club. Often, though, the items available through buying clubs—artisan cheese and heirloom varieties of certain fruits and vegetables—are not as readily available elsewhere.

KOL Foods, for instance, is an example of the unusual food offerings available through buying clubs. It is one of the few, organic kosher meat venues around. It is based in the Washington, DC, area, but has buying clubs in various locations, including San Francisco and Chicago. It ships all its meats to customers, but buying clubs can take advantage of reduced shipping rates because of the bulk purchases.

Food Co-ops. At food cooperatives or co-ops, members work and typically enjoy lower prices and higher quality food, including organic products. Typically, members pay a membership fee and work regularly—often several hours every few weeks—in the co-op, which keeps the prices down. There are more than twenty-nine thousand co-ops in the United States, with about three hundred fifty million co-op members, according to the National Cooperative Grocers Association (NCGA).

Co-ops are committed to local agriculture, having an average of 157 relationships with different local farmers, according to the NCGA. The average co-op purchases about 20 percent of products in the store from local sources. Typically, 82 percent of the produce and 48 percent of other grocery items are organic, notes NCGA. In addition, 89 percent of meat sold at co-ops is sustainably raised, and 75 percent of co-ops have product policies that restrict certain ingredients, such as genetically modified products and high fructose corn syrup, according to NCGA.

For instance, the Park Slope Food Co-op, founded in 1973 in Brooklyn, New York, offers local, organic, and conventionally grown produce; pasture-raised and grass-fed meat; free-range, organic, and kosher poultry; fair-traded chocolate and coffee; wild and sustainably farmed fish; supplements and vitamins; imported and artisan cheese; freshly baked bread; bulk grains and spices; and even environmentally safe cleaning supplies. The Co-op has found that its members save between 20 percent and 40 percent on their weekly grocery bill.

In addition, co-ops are committed to sustainability. The NCGA says that co-ops recycle 96 percent of the cardboard used, 74 percent of food waste, and 81 percent of plastics. Compare that with the stats for conventional grocers: 91 percent, 36 percent, and 29 percent, respectively. Co-ops also focus on lowering their energy use and carbon footprint, according to the NCGA.

Trend in Shopper Profiles

Over the past few years, research has found that Latinos and Asian Americans are more interested in organic foods than Caucasians or than the general US population, according to the Hartman Group. In 2009, the OTA found that more than half of surveyed Latinos choose organic foods to improve their health and the environment and to support farmers. And Latinos turn to organic food particularly when they have young children. Almost two out of every three Latino parents with a child under age ten (65 percent) buy organic—and more than half (57 percent) use organic food daily, according to the Hartman Group. By contrast, Latinos without young children have much less interest in avoiding GMOs and pesticides; only 17 percent of this population chooses organic food. This trend is not surprising when you consider that Latinos place a great deal of emphasis on family and that their "traditional" foods are organic.

Experts expect that this trend will continue as the number of Latinos increases in the United States. According to the US Census Bureau, there were 52 million Latinos in the United States as of July 1, 2011, making them the nation's largest ethnic minority. Over the previous year, the population grew 2.5 percent, and the Census Bureau estimates that, by 2050, there will be about 132.8 million Latinos in the United States.

Asian Americans are showing interest in organic foods as well. In an article published in *Pacific Citizen Magazine* in 2011, the OTA described Asian Americans as "an emerging market" in the organic arena. Again, demographics will play a role. Like the Latino population, the Asian American population is growing, too. The 2010 census estimated that there were 17.3 million Asians in the United States, representing about 5.6 percent of the US population. The US Census Bureau estimates that there will be approximately 40.6 million Asian Americans in the United States in 2050.

As the Latino and Asian American populations rise, and as these populations become more and more interested in organic food, their purchases may well have a broader effect on the American agricultural scene.

Mandatory Labeling

To label or not to label, that is the question. And a very controversial question it is, at least in the United States. (Elsewhere, such as in Europe, Japan, Australia, New Zealand, labeling GMO foods is quite commonplace.) Mandatory labeling has been proposed, and rejected, in more than a dozen US states and localities coast to coast, most recently in California, where it was nixed by a narrow margin. The contentious nature of the polls and votes suggests that we can expect this issue to continue to be hotly contested.

People in favor of mandatory labeling have a simple basic argument: We have the right to know what is in our food. With that information, we can make informed decisions about what we do—and do not—want to put into our bodies. The concern is particularly compelling for ingredients known to be carcinogenic or otherwise dangerous. Proponents argue that there haven't been enough studies done assessing the safety of GMO food, so people should be able to make their own, educated choices about what they want to eat and serve to their children. Surveys suggest that many Americans hold this opinion, though apparently not enough to pass a bill in any of the states or localities that have proposed it. However, businesses are paying attention. Whole Foods (see page 142) plans to have complete transparency about GMOs in its food by the year 2018.

Those opposed to mandatory labeling of GMO ingredients point out the expense and logistical difficulties of the undertaking. For instance, the storage, processing, and transportation components of the US food system cannot currently accommodate separation of GMO and traditional products. Not only that, but there would be additional costs associated with labeling, including testing the food items or extensive recordkeeping of the seed source, field location, harvest, transport, and storage process; as of this writing, there has been no study to suggest a dollar figure for all this. There's worry about the simplest things, like a bit of unwanted GMO seed or plant blowing from one farmer's field to another. In short, opponents of mandatory labeling are concerned that the costs of mandatory labeling outweigh the benefits.

In addition, opponents of mandatory labeling have logistical concerns. It is, for instance, unclear precisely what items or processes would require labeling, or how much of those particular ingredients would need to be mentioned; some countries have placed the threshold at less than 1 percent, while others have put it at 5 percent. Opponents of mandatory labeling also point out that in other countries, retailers have generally taken GMO items off their shelves, rather than provide additional customer choice, according to the Colorado State University. Opponents of mandatory labeling also claim that there has been no significant difference found between GMO and conventional foods in terms of health concerns. Customers who want to avoid GMO ingredients, these people suggest, can always just buy USDA-certified organic foods.

In short, this is a highly controversial issue and one that has not been resolved by the many polls and elections trying to decide it. We can certainly expect to see this issue come back again and again.

Non-GMO Project

For some, going organic isn't careful enough. Some people worry that the USDA-certified organic label isn't enough to keep them safe from genetically modified organisms. So they have been turning to another certification system, called the Non-GMO Project. When you buy USDA-certified organic foods, the US federal government certifies that there are no GMOs in the food. However, according to the Non-GMO Project, organic certification does not require GMO testing, so there remains a small possibility that there might be GMOs hidden inside the food.

The Non-GMO Project, a not-for-profit organization, started in 2003 in Berkeley, California, at a neighborhood natural foods store. The first store joined with several others to establish a consistent definition of "non-GMO." Today, the Non-GMO Project offers the only third-party verification and labeling for non-GMO food and products in North America. The Non-GMO Project labels foods as "Non-GMO Project Verified" when they pass ongoing evaluation—an annual audit and on-site inspections. The organization uses a threshold similar to the EU, of 0.9

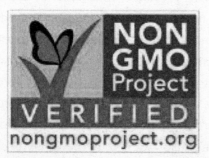

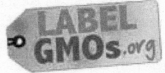

percent, where any product containing more than 0.9 percent genetically modified material must be labeled. It is working with Whole Foods in their GMO transparency initiative.

The Non-GMO Project is most concerned about "high-risk" products, namely: alfalfa, canola, corn, cotton, papaya, soy, sugar beets, zucchini, and yellow summer squash. The project also keeps a close eye on products that derive from these ingredients: amino acids, Aspartame, ascorbic acid, sodium ascorbate, vitamin C, citric acid, sodium citrate, ethanol, flavorings (both "natural" and "artificial"), high-fructose corn syrup, hydrolyzed vegetable protein, lactic acid, maltodextrins, molasses, monosodium glutamate, sucrose, textured vegetable protein (TVP), xanthan gum, vitamins, and yeast products.

The Project is aided in its efforts by Food Chain Global Advisors, a company with expertise in biotechnology, molecular biology, genetics, and other approaches to analyzing traceability and identity preservation. Non-GMO Project-verified products are gaining in popularity, the organization notes. Specifically, sales of these products are growing by 27 percent and reached $450 million in 2010.

Gaining Ground Around the Globe

GMOs are controversial not just in the United States, but all around the world. Just as in the United States, the rules and laws governing production and labeling are constantly changing and evolving, as is public opinion. It can be hard to keep up.

Some countries, such as Canada, Mexico, and China, embrace GMOs, seeing them as a gift of scientific research and the best way to alleviate world hunger for a growing population. Other countries see GMOs as the scourge of the earth, responsible for environmental, moral, and medical ills; Zimbabwe, Malawi, and Mozambique, for instance, refused foreign food aid during a drought because it contained genetically modified organisms.

Organic agricultural land and farms, as well as the global market continued to grow during 2009, as documented in the 2011 edition of the

World of Organic Agriculture, from the Research Institute of Organic Agriculture (FiBL) and the International Federation of Organic Agriculture Movements (IFOAM). According to the latest FiBL/IFOAM survey on certified organic agriculture worldwide, there are 37.2 million hectares of organic agricultural land worldwide. As of 2011, 0.9 percent of the world's agricultural land is organic. Compared with the previous survey, with data from 2008, organic land increased by two million hectares, or 6 percent. Growth was strongest in Europe, where the area increased by almost one million hectares.

As of 2009, the countries with the largest markets for organic food are the United States, Germany, and France; the highest per capita consumption of organic foods are Denmark, Switzerland, and Austria, according to the *World of Organic Agriculture* report.

As difficult as it is to predict the future of genetically modified organisms in our own country, it is even harder to figure out what is happening—and what is going to happen—in other parts of the world. Here's a quick sense of what other countries are thinking about and doing in regard to genetically modified foods.

The European Union (EU)

As of the end of 2010, Europe had approximately 10 million hectares of organic producers, according FiBL/IFOAM; this represents about a quarter (27 percent) of worldwide organic land. The countries with the greatest organic agricultural area are Spain (1.5 million hectares), Italy (1.1 million hectares), and Germany (.99 million hectares), notes FiBL/FOAM.

The European Union has set up a legal framework to regulate GMO food and animal feed throughout the EU. Beyond the basic guidelines, an individual country can prohibit use or sale of a particular GMO under a "safeguard clause." So far, according to the European Commission, six EU states have applied safeguard clauses: Austria, France, Greece, Hungary, Germany, and Luxembourg. According to GMO Compass, a website funded by the European Union, the only GMO currently grown in its member countries is Bt corn. Here are some more specifics on the countries:

- **Austria**: In 2010, more than 19 percent of the country's agricultural area was organic, according to FiBL/FOAM. That ranks it second in relative hectares, next to Lichtenstein. It was one of the first countries worldwide to set official guidelines for organic farming. Organic foods are sold in supermarket chains and specialty stores; studies show that 20 percent of the consumers buy 80 percent of the organic food, according to FiBL/FOAM.

- **Czech Republic**: Bt corn has been grown here since 2005, according to GMO Compass.

- **Finland**: Organically managed land is a small yet growing force in Finland, according to FiBL/FOAM. It represented 1 percent of agricultural land in 1989, but by 2008, it was almost 7 percent. According to GMO Compass, the Finnish government and citizens are more accepting of genetically modified crops than the rest of the EU.

- **Germany**: The German public is also opposed to GMOs, but many politicians support biotechnology, notes GMO Compass. Bt corn has been grown commercially since 2004, and in 2005, it represented 0.1 percent of the country's total corn production.

- **Great Britain**: The UK government has an accepting but cautious approach toward GMO crops. There won't be any commercially grown genetically modified foods, though, until the country has developed legal guidelines for the coexistence of GMO and non-GMO crops, according to GMO Compass. FiBL/FOAM notes that the organic market in the UK relies on a small but devoted core of consumers, a third of whom are manual and casual workers, pensioners, students, and people receiving public assistance.

- **Greece**: Greek citizens are also opposed to GMOs, and even EU-approved crops are banned in the country, according to GMO

Compass. Most regions are GMO-free, and there are currently no genetically modified crops being grown in Greece.

- **The Netherlands**: More hospitable than most of the EU to the idea of genetically modified organisms, the Netherlands is the first EU country to establish legal guidelines for the coexistence of GMO and non-GMO crops, according to GMO Compass. But there are still no GMO crops planted, notes GMO Compass.

- **Portugal**: As with the Czech Republic, Bt corn has been grown here since 2005, according to GMO Compass.

- **Spain**: This country has more experience with Bt corn than anywhere else in the EU; it has been grown commercially here since 1988. Estimates place Bt corn production at 25 percent of total corn produced in Spain. At the same time, organic acreage increased by 10 percent in 2011, reaching a total of 1.6 million hectares or 6.5 percent of the agricultural land, according to FiBL/FOAM.

- **Turkey**: No GMO crops have been approved for food, but the country has approved sixteen GMO soybean and corn plants for feed use.

Australia and New Zealand

Food Standards Australia New Zealand (FSANZ), part of the Australian government, develops food standards for both Australia and New Zealand. FSANZ states that it will not approve a genetically modified food unless it is safe to eat. Thus far, several varieties have been approved of GMO canola, corn, soybean, rice, lucerne, wheat, cotton, sugar beet, and potato. As of 2009, Australian and Tasmanian farmers are lagging the world in conversion to organic, according to John Paull, PhD.[91]

- **Australia**: As of the end of 2008-09, there were a total of 2,986 certified organic operators in Australia, representing about 1.6 percent of all farming operations in Australia. The farmers work 12,001,724 hectares, the largest amount of certified organic farmland in the world. Most people start with organic fruits and vegetables before moving on to other organic products, and the majority buy organic food at their local supermarkets (more than 60 percent). In addition, there has also been a strong growth in farmers' markets.

- **New Zealand:** New Zealanders bought a total of 315 million NZ$ of domestic organic products in 2010, according to the New Zealand Organic Report 2010, which was commissioned by OANZ and prepared by the University of Otago. The country also produced an additional 170 million NZ $ (94 million euros) for export. As of the time of the report, New Zealand had 1,145 certified organic farmers, working on more than 124,000 hectares of land.[92]

North America

In general, North America is relatively accepting of genetically modified organisms. The United States is in good company, as it were.

- **Mexico**: One of the "founding" countries of GMO, Mexico has been growing Bt corn since 1996, with the rate of GMO crops doubling between 2010 and 2011, reaching 175,000 hectares of genetically modified crops, according to the International Service for the Acquisition of Agri-Biotech Applications (ISAAA). GMO soybean crops are concentrated in three states: Peninsula (which planted 9,042 hectares); Tamaulipas (1,647 hectares); and Chiapas (3,491 hectares).
- **Canada**: Health Canada and the Canadian Food Inspection Agency (CFIA) require product developers to gain approval for sale in Canada. As of 2012, according to Health Canada, more than seventy GMO foods have been approved for sale in Canada. On November 19, 2012, the Council of Saanich, British Columbia, voted unanimously against the use of genetically modified seed crops within the District. Saanich is the seventh BC municipality to ban GM seed crops, joining Powell River, Nelson, New Denver,

Kaslo, Rossland, and Richmond, according to the Canada Organic Trade Association.

Asia

In 2010, Asia planted about 2.8 million hectares of organic land, or roughly 7 percent of the world's agricultural land, according to FiBL/FOAM. Between 2009 and 2010, there was a decrease in organic farming, led by China and India. Some countries—China, Japan, the Philippines, South Korea, and Taiwan specifically—use third-party certified organic labeling, according to FiBL/FOAM. As of 2005, several Asian countries have approved imports, others have approved field testing, and some have approved growing GMO crops commercially. Japan, China, Australia, India, and Indonesia, notes GMO Compass, have granted all three types of approvals.

- **China**: The government has assigned high priority to development of biotechnology, according to the International Service for the Acquisition of Agri-Biotech Applications (ISAAA). Total increase in GMO crops in 2011 was 11 percent; China grew 2 percent of the world's biotech, at 160 million hectares. For instance, Bt cotton represented 71.5 percent of all cotton grown in China in 2011, or about 3.9 million hectares. Other GMO crops planted commercially were poplar, sweet peppers, tomatoes, and papaya, notes ISAAA.
- **India**: While 88 percent of Indian farmers plant GMO crops, there remains strong opposition to genetically modified foods, according to ISAAA. Bt cotton is growing astronomically; plantings reached 10.6 million hectares or 88 percent of the country's cotton crop, up from 9.4 million hectares (13 percent) in 2010. Cotton is the only GMO currently planted in India, but the public sector is working on genetically engineered brinjal, groundnut, mustard, papaya, potato, rice, sorghum, sugar cane, tomato, and watermelon, while the private sector is developing brinjal, cabbage, cauliflower, cotton, maize, okra, rice, and tomato. At the

same time, India is one of the three countries in the world with the most organic producers, 677, 257 as of 2009, according to FiBL/ FOAM.

- **Japan**: Taking a "scientific-based risk assessment" approach to GMO assessment, Japan stands somewhere between the EU's stringent rules on labeling and the United States' less careful approach. Japan feels that it is impossible to completely separate dust and admixtures from genetically modified and traditionally grown crops, according to the Gianinni Foundation of Agricultural Economics at the University of California.

- **Pakistan**: In 2010, Pakistan became the thirteenth country in the world to plant GMO cotton, and now the government and Pakistan Central Cotton Committee (PCCC) are counting on GMO crops to help it reach its cotton-planting target of 19.1 million bales by 2015, according to the ISAAA. They're on their way, qualifying as the fourth-largest cotton producer in the world after China, India, and the United States.

- **Philippines**: This country achieved a biotech "megacountry status" in 2004, according to the ISAAA, by planting more than 50,000 hectares of GMO corn. Since then, the Philippine commitment to GMO corn has continued to grow, planting 644,000 hectares in 2011.The country is also testing out genetically modified rice, eggplant, papaya, cotton, and sweet potato, according to the ISAAA.

Africa

Africa as a whole has its doubts about GMO crops. During the drought of 2002-2003, notes the United Nations Environment Programme, several countries rejected GMO food aid. They were concerned about the overall implications for human and environmental health, as well as concern for future, private sector-led research and ethical issues. Zimbabwe, Malawi, and Mozambique refused to accept GMO food aid unless it was milled, while Lesotho and Swaziland authorized distribution of nonmilled GMO food aid, warning the public that it should be used only for consumption, not for cultivation. In 2004, Angola and Sudan introduced restrictions on GMO food aid. According to FiBL/FOAM, African policy makers are beginning to realize the role that organic food can make in alleviating food insecurity, poverty, and climate change across the continent.

- **Egypt**: The country consumes plenty of GMO foods, including corn and soybeans, but doesn't grow any locally, as of 2009, according to the USDA Foreign Agricultural Service. They've planted GMO corn and cotton in several regions throughout the country to conduct field trials and are conducting research on potatoes, squash, wheat, and rice.
- **South Africa**: The Consumer Protection Act of 2008 requires labeling of genetically modified crops. And there are plenty to label, according to the ISAAA. South Africa currently plants Bt corn, Bt wheat, and GMO wheat. It has granted 348 GMO permits in 2010 and another 173 from January to July 2011.
- **Zimbabwe**: The country has banned imports of GMO crop seeds and products, according to the *Zimbabwean*. But the topic is still controversial within the government. The Minister of Agriculture says that GMOs are toxic, while the Prime Minister maintains that there is no scientific proof of that. The country has accepted GMO food aid, provided it has already been milled, according to the United Nations Environment Programme.

South America

In 2010, Latin America had approximately 8.4 million hectares of organic farmland, according to FiBL/FOAM. This is about 23 percent of the world's organic farmland and 1.4 percent of the region's agricultural land. Argentina, Brazil, and Uruguay lead the way in organic farmland, but 85 percent of what is produced heads to the United States, Europe, and Japan. According to FiBL/FOAM, the organic movement anticipates more acceptance of organic food for domestic use over the coming years.

- **Argentina**: Maintaining its place as the third-largest GMO grower in the world, Argentina farmed 23.7 million hectares with GMO crops, which is about 15 percent of the global total. They planted 19.1 million hectares of GMO soybean, 3.9 million hectares of GMO corn, and 0.7 million hectares of genetically modified cotton. According to the ISAAA, there are twenty-one GMO crops approved for planting in Argentina. But Argentina's story is not only GMO. It is also one of the three countries in the world with the most organic agricultural land, and also one of the three with the greatest gains in farming organic land, notes FiBL/ FOAM, planting 4.2 million hectares of organic farmland.
- **Brazil**: The second-largest grower of GMO crops in the world, next to the United States, Brazil grew 30.3 million hectares of biotech crops or 75 percent of soybean, corn, and cotton, up from 4.9 million hectares (19 percent) in 2010; this represents the largest increase in any country in the world, according to the ISAAA. And they're not stopping there. Brazil approved eight GMO crops in 2010 and another six in the first ten months of 2011—the country with the fastest approval rate for biotech crops in the world, according to ISAAA. The country also plants 1.8 million hectares of organic farmland, notes FiBL/FOAM.
- **Peru**: A ten-year ban of genetically modified organisms came into effect in 2012, according to the *Andean Air Mail and Peruvian Times*. The ban is intended to protect Peru's organic and native products, which are being exported more and more.

Bear in mind that the agricultural industry changes constantly within the United States. The same is true around the world. It is interesting to see how differently people view the issues of GMOs—which include having enough food, maintaining our health, our right to know what we are buying, and government regulation—and to see that whether you are in Zimbabwe or Cleveland, Ohio, people are struggling with the same concerns: How do we best feed ourselves and our families?

Whole Foods Market

Year Founded: 1980

   Products: Just about everything you'd need.

   Where to Buy: More than 340 stores in 39 states as well as the UK and Canada.

Whole Foods has announced that by 2018, it will have complete transparency about GMOs. All products sold in the United States or Canada will be labeled if they contain genetically modified organisms. This makes it the first national grocery chain to set a deadline for GMO transparency.

"We have always believed that quality and transparency are inseparable and that providing detailed information about the products we offer...is part of satisfying and delighting the millions of people who place their trust in Whole Foods Market each day," said A.C. Gallo, president of Whole Foods Market. "This bold task will encourage manufacturers to ask deeper questions about ingredients, and it will help us provide greater transparency about the products we sell so our customers can be empowered to make informed decisions about the foods that are best for them."

At the same time, Whole Foods is increasing its support of certified organic foods. The national supermarket chain currently sells 3,300 Non-GMO Project verified products from 250 brands, as well as its own private label of organic food, 365 Everyday Value® food products.

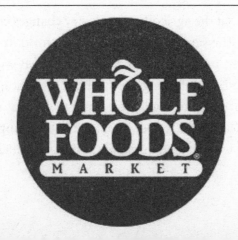

Producers You Can Trust

PRODUCERS ENDORSED BY THE CORNUCOPIA INSTITUTE

The Cornucopia Institute, a nonprofit farm policy research group, acts as an organic industry watchdog. It has published a number of comprehensive reports scrutinizing segments of the organic market (such as dairy products, soy foods, eggs, and cereal). Its goal is to separate faux organic (factory farms, Chinese imports) from authentic organic food. In addition, the Cornucopia Institute website includes scorecards rating organic brands, which enables consumers and wholesale buyers to make discerning marketplace decisions.

Please note that the following list, taken from their website, is constantly changing. For the most up-to-date list of suppliers, visit their website at www.cornucopia.org.

Soy Producers

California
House Foods, Los Angeles
Tofu Shop, Arcata
Whole Soy, San Francisco
Wildwood, Fullerton

Canada
Green Cuisine, Victoria
Pete's Tofu, Vancouver, B.C.
Unisoya, Quebec

Illinois
Lifeway, Morton Grove

Kansas
Central Soy Foods, Lawrence

Massachusetts
Nasoya, Ayer
Vitasoy, Ayer

Minnesota
Eden Foods, Clinton

New Hampshire
O'Soy, Londonderry

New York
Soy Boy, Rochester

North Carolina
Harris Teeter, Private Label,
    Matthews
Miso Master, Asheville

Ohio
Baby's Only Organic, Columbus

Oregon
Nancy's, Eugene
Turfurky, Hood River

Pennsylvania
Fresh Tofu, Allentown

Tennessee
FarmSoy, Summerton

Texas
365, Austin

Vermont
Rhapsody Natural Foods, Montpelier
Twin Oaks, Louisa
Vermont Soya, Hardwick

Virginia
Sunergia, Charlottesville

Washington
Small Planet, Newport

Wisconsin
Organic Valley, La Farge

Eggs

California
Alexandre Kids, Crescent City
Amsterdam Organics, Winton
Burroughs Family Farms Eggs,
    Denair

Clover Organic Farms, Petaluma
Lazy 69 Ranch, Round Mountain
Organic Pastures, Fresno
St. John Family Farm, Orland

Colorado
Grant Family Farms, Wellington

Connecticut
Turtle Ledge Farm, Hampton

Florida
Bee Heaven Farm, Homestead
PNS Farms, Miami

Iowa
Farmer's Hen House, Kalona

Maine
Happy Town Farm, Orland
One Drop Farm, Cornville
Village Farm, Freedom

Massachusetts
Born Free, Watertown
Old Friends Farm, Amherst
Stony Book Valley Farm, Granby

Michigan
Krause Farm, Engadine

Minnesota
Schultz Eggs, Owatonna

Missouri
Green Hills Harvest

Montana
Mission Mountain, Ronan

Nebraska
Common Good Farm, Raymond
Mosel Eggs, Page

New Hampshire
Pete & Gerry's, Monroe

New York
Handsome Brook Farm, Franklin
Kingbird Farm, Berkshire
Neversink Farm, Claryville
Windy Ridge Natural Farms,
  Alfred

Ohio
Green Field Farms, Fredericksburg
Morning Sun Farm, West
  Alexandria

Oregon
Phoenix Egg Farm, Portland
WAC Eggs, Champoeg

Pennsylvania
B Dabler, Greencastle
Giving Nature, Holicong
Misera Family Farm, Butler

Nature's Yoke, New Holland

Texas
World's Best Eggs, Eglin
Vital Farms, Austin

Utah
First Frost Farm, Nibley

Vermont
Cleary Family Farm, Plainview
Doolittle Farm, Middlebury
Highfields Farm, Randolph
River Berry Farm, Fairfax

Virginia
Shenandoah Family Farms,
    Dayton

Washington
Hi Q Organic, Sedro Woolley
Misty Meadows Farm, Everson
Skagit River Ranch, Sedro Woolley
Stiebrs, Yelm
Trout Lake Abbey, Trout Lake
Wilcox Farms, Roy

Wisconsin
Coon Creek, Mondovi
Dreamfarm, Cross Plains
Egg Innovations, Port Washington
Green Pastures Poultry, Cashton
Milo's Organic, Bonduel
New Century, Shullsberg

Organic Valley, LaFarge
Whispering Spruce, LaFarge

Dairy

California
Clover Organic Farms, Petaluma
Cowgirl Creamery, Point Reyes
    Station
Food Maxx (Sunnyside Farms),
    Stockton
Loleta Cheese, Loleta
Natural Choice, Oxnard
Organic Pastures Dairy Company,
    Fresno
Potter Family Farms, Visalia
Raley's, Nob Hill, Bel Air, Food
Sierra Nevada Cheese Company,
    Willows
Source (Sunnyside Farms) ,
Stockton
Straus Family Creamery, Marshall
Stremicks (Heritage-Foods), Santa Ana
Wallaby Yogurt, Napa, CA (yogurt,
    ice cream)

Colorado
Boulder Ice Cream, Boulder

Delaware
This Land is Your Land,
    Wilmington

Idaho
Glanbia Falls, Twin Falls

Illinois
Heavenly Organics, Inc., Fairfield
Lifeway, Morton Grove
Similac (Abbott Laboratories),
  Abbott Park

Indiana
Traders Point Farms, Zionsville

Iowa
Cultural Revolution (Kalona
  Organics), Kalona
HyVee 4, West Des Moines
Kalona Supernatural, Wellman
Radiance Dairy, Fairfield

Maine
MOO Maine's Own Organic Milk,
  Augusta

Minnesota
Cedar Summit Dairy, New Prague
Helios, Centre
Hope Creamery, Hope
PastureLand, Dodge Center

Missouri
Fluid Green Hills Harvest, Purdin

New Hampshire
Stonyfield (yogurt, fluid milk),
  Londonderry

New Jersey
Amish Country Farms, Totowa

Green and Black's Organic-USA,
  Parsippany
Harris Teeter, Carlstadt
Pure Indian Foods, Lawrenceville

New Mexico
Coonridge Dairy, Coonridge

New York
Evans Farmhouse Creamery,
  Norwich
Hawthorne Valley Farm, Ghent
Perry's Ice Cream, Akron
Sky Top Farms, Bronx
Upstate Farms, Buffalo
Wegmans Food Markets,
  Rochester

Ohio
Green Field Farms, Fredericksburg
Nature's One, Columbus

Oregon
Julie's (Oregon Ice Cream), Eugene
Nancy's Springfield Dairy, Eugene

Pennsylvania
Bridge View Dairy, Oxford
Hails Family Farm, Wyalusing
Kimberton Hills, Phoenixville
Natural by Nature, West Grove
Seven Stars, Phoenixville
Trickling Springs Creamery,
  Chambersberg

South Carolina
Ingles Markets (Harvest Farms),
  Black Mountain

Texas
Whole Foods Markets (365
  organic), Austin

Vermont
Animal Farm, Orwell
Ben and Jerry's, South Burlingon
Butterworks Farm, Westfield
Strafford Organic Creamery,
  Strafford
Thistle Hill Farm, North Pomfret

Washington
Fresh Breeze Organic Dairy,
  Lynden

Yami Organic (Auburn Dairy),
  Auburn

Wisconsin
Castle Rock Farms, Osseo
Cedar Grove Cheese, Plain
Crystal Ball Farms, Osceola
Organic Creamery (DCI Cheese),
  Sun Prairie
Organic Valley (CROPP), La Farge
Sassy Cow Creamery, Columbus
Scenic Central Milk Prod. Co-op,
  Prairie Du Sac
Sibby Farm, Westby
Westby Cooperative Creamery,
  Westby
Wisconsin Organics, Thorp

BEEF AND RUMINANT PRODUCERS ENDORSED BY THE AMERICAN GRASSFED ASSOCIATION

The American Grassfed Association defines grassfed products from ruminants, including cattle, bison, goats, and sheep, as those food products from animals that have eaten nothing but their mother's milk and fresh grass or grass-type hay from their birth. The organization's website lists all certified producers by state and alphabetically.

Once again, this list is constantly changing, so be sure to visit their site at www.americangrassfed.org for the current list.

Alabama
Hastings Farms, Bay Minette
Miller Farms, Delta

Arizona
Rose Ranches, Payson

California
Bear Valley River Beef, Ferndale
Brandon Natural Beef, San Francisco
Ferndale Farms, Ferndale
Holding Ranch, Montague
Homegrown Meats / Mendenhall Ranch, La Jolla
Leftcoast Grassfed, Pescadero
Marin Sun Farms, San Francisco
Markegard Family Grass-Fed, San Gregorio
Morris Grassfed, San Juan Bautista
Old Creek Ranch, Cayucos
Paradise Valley Beef, Fairfield
Potter 8 Ranch, Loyalton
Rabb Cattle Co., Woodlake
Scott River Ranch, Etna
Sierra Lands Beef, Prather
Striking A Livestock, Vina
True Grass Farms-Conlan Ranches California, Valley Ford

Colorado
Canyon of The Ancients Guest Ranch, Cortez
Flying B Bar Ranch, Strasburg

James Ranch, Durango
KDL. Ranch, Kiowa
KW Farms, Alamosa
Lasater Grassland Beef, Matheson
Oswald Cattle Co / Back Country Beef, Cotopaxi
Our Pastures 100% Grassfed Beef Company, Denver
Pharo Cattle Company, Cheyenne Wells
Princess Beef, Hotchkiss
Rocky Plains, LLP, Dacono
Salazar Natural Meats, Manassa
Sangre's Best Grass Fed Beef, Westcliffe
Shining Horizons Land Management, San Luis
Sun Prairie Beef, Yuma
Sylvan Dale Guest Ranch, Loveland
Windsor Dairy, Windsor

Connecticut
JW Beef, Stonington
JW Beef/Stonington Lowlines, Stonington
Stuart Family Farm, Bridgewater

Florida
Pasture Prime Family Farm, Summerfield
Rocking T Ranch, Laurel Hill
Sampson Family Farm, Live Oak

Georgia

Cooke Cattle Company, Atlanta
Double AJ Farms, LLC, Davisboro
Hunter Cattle Company, Brooklet
Hunter Cattle Company, Brooklet
Koinonia Farm, Americus
Savannah River Farms, Sylvania
Wagon Wheel Ranch, Watkinsville
White Oak Pastures, Bluffton

Idaho

Lau Family Farm, LLC, Soda
   Springs
Lava Lake Lamb, Hailey

Illinois

Flying S Beef, Palestine
Harvest Hills Farm, Hanover
Homestead Harvests, Heyworth
Plum River Farm, Pearl City
Sangamon Valley Cattle Co.,
   Pleasant Plains

Indiana

Hoosier Grassfed Beef, Attica
The Swiss Connection, Clay City
Traders Point Creamery, Zionsville
Traders Point Farm Organics,
   Zionsville

Kansas

Chapman Creek Cattle Co.,
   Topeka
JaKo, Inc., Hutchinson

Kentucky

Ashbourne Farms, La Grange
Brookview Farm Dba Brookview
   Beef, Winchester
Colcord Farm, Paris

Louisiana

Gardner Ranch, Sunset
Gonsoulin Land and Cattle, LLC,
   New Iberia

Maryland

KOL Foods, Silver Spring
West Wind Farm, Bethesda
Whitmore Farm, Emmitsburg

Michigan

Garrett Cattle Company, Mt
   Pleasant

Mississippi

Amber Grassfed Beef, Hickory

Missouri

7 Springs Farm, Mansfield
American GrassFed Beef, Doni-
   phan
Angel Acres Farm, LLC, Bland
Hewkin Farms And Cattle LLC,
   Cuba
Ozarks Natural Beef, Rogersville
Stropes RSK Farm, Chilhowee
Sunrise Pastures/The Masters
   Ranch, Laclede

Swope Cattle Company, Cuba

Montana
Ferry Creek Ranch, Livingston
La Cense Beef, LLC, Dillon

Nebraska
Boettcher Organics, Bassett
Straight Arrow Bison Ranch,
　Broken Bow

New Jersey
7th Heaven Farm LLC, Tabernacle
Pure Indian Foods, Princeton
　Junction
Simply Grazin' LLC, Skillman

New Mexico
L6 Cattle Ranches, LLC, Corona
Moonbeam Ranch, Edgewood
Southwest Grassfed Livestock
　Alliance, Santa Fe
Taos Mountain Yak, LLC, Arroyo
　Seco

New York
Heydenrych Farms, Canajoharie
High Lonesome Farm, Cincin-
　natus
Lee Farms, Kent
Mack Brook Farm, Argyle

North Carolina
Delmar Farm Inc., Enfield

Hardrock Beef Cattle, Granite
　Falls
Hilltop Angus Farm, Mount
　Gilead
Little Creek Ranch, Liberty
Meadows Family Farms, Julian
Poplin Farms Inc., Albemarle
Proffitt Family Cattle Co., Kings
　Mountain
River Taw Farms LLC, Cherryville

Ohio
Kraut Creek Sheep & Cattle,
　Greenville
Spring Hill Farms, Newark
White Clover Farm, Hillsboro

Oklahoma
Aird M'Hor, Roff
Nitschke Natural Beef/Circle N
　Ranch, Waurika

Oregon
Carman Ranch, Wallowa
Foss Road Beef LLC, Nehalem
Happy Cow Farms, Inc., Dallas
Niche Meat Processor Assistance
　Network, Corvallis
Rudio Creek Ranch, Salem

Pennsylvania
JuJo Acres Farm, Loysville
Lil' Ponderosa Enterprises, Carlisle
WindSwept Farm, Ulster

South Dakota
Dakota Harvest Farm, Jefferson

Texas
A+S, Moulton
Adams Blackland Prairie, Ladonia
Arcadian Haven, Limited
  Company, Elgin
Bandera Grassland, Tarpley
Bar W.T. Ranch, Conroe
Bar J Grassfed Beef, Inc.,
  Coupland
Bonner Farm, Valley Spring
Burgundy Pasture Beef,
  Grandview
Crawley's Country Beef, LLC,
  Hubbard
Diamond N Ranch, Seminole
Eagle Catcher Farm & Ranch,
  Harlingen
F Bar Springs Ranch, Wichita Falls
Flying Cowgirls Ranch Products,
  Rosston
GrassField Beef, Hondo
Green Grass, Austin
J1 Ranch, Athens
Koch Ranches, Inc., San Antonio
L&B Cattle Company, LLC,
  Detroit
L&M Beef, Floresville
Lazy A Ranch, Bellville

Lovejoy Farm, Clifton
Madroño Ranch, Medina
Maggies Farm, Schulenburg
McCollum-Lemke Ranches,
  Mason
Perez L And M Ranch,
  Floresville
Red River Ranch, Clarksville
Shudde Ranch, Sabinal
Sabra Ranch, La Grange
TA Ranch, Perrin
Thunder Heart Bison, San Antonio
Watterson Ranch, Bastrop
Windfall Ranch, Lexington

Tennessee
Big B Ranch, Petersburg
Gourmet Pasture Beef, Springfield
Wildcat Ranch, McEwen

Vermont
Smith Maple Crest Farm LLC,
  Shrewsbury

Virginia
Riven Rock Farm, Monterey
Wolf Creek Farm, Wolftown

Washington
Aspen Hollow Sheep Station,
  Redmond

Grass Fed Beef - J. Hutton,
  Ellensburg
HolyCowGrassfed.Com, Wapato
Windy N Ranch, Ellensburg

West Virginia
Critton Creek Farm, Pawpaw

Wisconsin
Grass Point Farms, Thorp
Seven Seeds   Green
  Farm, Spring
V D B Organic Farms, Delavan

Notes

1   USDA, *Pesticide Data Program: Annual Summary, Calendar Year 2010,* May 2012, www.ams.usda.gov/AMSv1.0/getfile?dDocName=stel prdc5098550.

2   Eunmi Koh, Suthawan Charoenprasert, and Alyson E. Mitchell, "Effect of Organic and Conventional Cropping Systems on Ascorbic Acid, Vitamin C, Flavonoids, Nitrate, and Oxalate in 27 Varieties of Spinach (Spinacia oleracea L.)," *Journal of Agricultural and Food Chemistry* 60, no. 12 (2012): 3144–3150.

3   Alyson E. Mitchell, "A Comparison of the Nutrient and Phytochemical Content of Organic and Conventional Tomatoes and Peppers," (Power-Point slides for the *Organic Seed Alliance,* Portland, Oregon, January 11, 2006), mitchell.ucdavis.edu/OSA2006_Mitchell2.pdf.

4   Alyson E. Mitchell and Alexander W. Chassy, "Antioxidants and the Nutritional Quality of Organic Agriculture," mitchell.ucdavis.edu/Is%20 Organic%20Better.pdf.

5   A. G. Zwald and others, "Management practices and reported antimicrobial usage on conventional and organic dairy farms," *J Dairy Sci* 87, no. 1 (2004): 191-201, www.ncbi.nlm.nih.gov/pubmed/14765827.

6   William J. Cromie, "Growth Factor Raises Cancer Risk," *The Harvard University Gazette*, http://www.news.harvard.edu/gazette/1999/04.22/igf1.story.html.

7   Endogenous Hormones and Breast Cancer Collaborative Group and others, "Insulin-like growth factor 1 (IGF1), IGF binding protein 3 (IGFBP3), and breast cancer risk: pooled individual data analysis of 17 prospective studies," *Lancet Oncol* 11, no. 6 (2010): 530-42.

8   A. J. Price and others, "Insulin-like growth factor-I concentration and risk of prostate cancer: results from the European Prospective Investigation into Cancer and Nutrition," *Cancer Epidemiology, Biomarkers & Prevention* 21, no. 9: 1531–41, doi: 10.1158/1055-9965.EPI-12-0481-T.

9   Karen Collins, "Organic milk: Are the benefits worth the cost?" NBCNews.com, August 25, 2006, http://www.msnbc.msn.com/id/14458802/ns/health-diet_and_nutrition/t/organic-milk-are-benefits-worth-cost/#.UL4YWuSOQgo.

10   Joel Forman, Janet Silverstein Committee on Nutrition, and Council on Environmental Health, "Organic Foods: Health and Environmental Advantages and Disadvantages," *Pediatrics* (2012): e1406-e1416, pediatrics.aappublications.org/content/early/2012/10/15/peds.2012-2579.full.pdf+html.

11   A. P. Raun and R. L. Preston, "History of diethylstilbestrol use in cattle," *American Society of Animal Science* (2002), http://www.asas.org/docs/publications/raunhist.pdf?sfvrsn=0.

12   A. L. Herbst, H. Ulfelder, and D. C. Poskanzer, "Adenocarcinoma of the Vagina. Association of maternal stilbestrol therapy with tumor appearance in young women," *N Engl J Med* 284, no. 15 (1971): 878-81, www.ncbi.nlm.nih.gov/pubmed/5549830.

13   Raun and Preston, "History of diethylstilbestrol."

14   Leticia M. Diaz, "Hormone replacement therapy, or just eat more meat: the technological hare vs. the regulatory tortoise," *Boston College Environmental Affairs Law Review* 27, no. 3 (2000), lawdigitalcommons.bc.edu/ealr/vol27/iss3/3.

15 Ellin Doyle, "Human Safety of Hormone Implants Used to Promote Growth in Cattle," Food Research Institute, U of Wisconsin (2000), fri. wisc.edu/docs/pdf/hormone.pdf.

16 Diaz, "Hormone replacement therapy."

17 Ibid.

18 Andrew E. Waters and others, "Multidrug-resistant Staphylococcus aureus in US meat and poultry," Clinical Infectious Diseases 52, no. 10 (2011): 1227-1230.

19 "Nationwide study finds US meat and poultry is widely contaminated," the Translational Genomics Research Institute, accessed March 20, 2013, http://www.eurekalert.org/pub_releases/2011-04/ttgr-nsf041311.php.

20 US Dept. of Health and Human Services, Guidance for Industry: The Judicious Use of Medically Important Antimicrobial Drugs in Food-Producing Animals, April 13, 2012, http://www.fda.gov/downloads/AnimalVeterinary/GuidanceComplianceEnforcement/GuidanceforIndustry/UCM216936.pdf.

21 S. Sarasua and D. A. Savitz, "Cured and broiled meat consumption in relation to childhood cancer: Denver, Colorado (United States)," Cancer Causes and Control 5, no. 2 (1994): 141-8, www.ncbi.nlm.nih.gov/pubmed/8167261.

22 John M. Peters and others, "Processed meats and risk of childhood leukemia (California, USA)," Cancer Causes and Control 5 (1994): 195-202, www.missclasses.com/mp3s/Prize%20CD%202010/Previous%20years/hot%20dogs/leukemia.pdf.

23 Ute Nothlings and others, "Meat and fat intake as risk factors for pancreatic cancer: The Multiethnic Cohort Study," JNCI 97, no. 19 (2005): 1458-1465, doi: 10.1093/jnci/dji292.

24 R. Sinha and others, "Meat intake and mortality: a prospective study of over half a million people," Arch Intern Med 169, no. 6 (2009): 562-71.

25 "AICR Statement: Hot Dogs and Cancer Risk," American Institute for Cancer Research, July 22, 2009, http://preventcancer.aicr.org/site/News2 ?page=NewsArticle&id=15642&news_iv_ctrl=0&abbr=pr_.

26 Doris Stanley, "Irradiation helps keep meat safe," *Agricultural Research* (1995), http://www.ars.usda.gov/is/ar/archive/nov95/irradiation1195. htm?pf=.

27 C. A. Daley and others, "A review of fatty acid profiles and antioxidant content in grass-fed and grain-fed beef," *Nutr J.* 9, no. 10 (2010), http:// www.csuchico.edu/grassfedbeef/research/Review%20Grassfed%20 Beef%202010.pdf.

28 Sarah DiGregorio, "Battle of the Dishes: Grass-Fed, Local Steak Versus Supermarket Steak," *The Village Voice,* November 5, 2009, http://blogs. villagevoice.com/forkintheroad/2009/11/battle_of_the_d_18.php

29 "Agricultural Policies Versus Health Policies," Physicians Committee for Responsible Medicine, accessed March 20, 2013, http://www.pcrm.org/ search/?cid=2466.

30 Chensheng Lu and others, "Organic diets significantly lower children's dietary exposure to organophosphorus pesticides," *Environ Health Perspect* 114, no. 2 (2006): 260–263.

31 Maryse F. Bouchard and others, "Attention-deficit/hyperactivity disorder and urinary metabolites of organophosphate pesticides," *Pediatrics* (2010), http://pediatrics.aappublications.org/content/ early/2010/05/17/peds.2009-3058.abstract.

32 M. F. Bouchard, "Prenatal Exposure to Organophosphate Pesticides and IQ in 7-Year-Old Children," *Environ Health Perspect* 119, no. 8 (2011): 1189-95.

33 S. M. Engel and others, "Prenatal exposure to organophosphates, paraoxonase 1, and cognitive development in childhood," *Environ Health Perspect* 119, no. 8 (2011): 1182-8.

34 Janie F. Shelton, Irva Hertz-Picciotto, and Isaac N. Pessah, "Tipping the balance of autism risk: potential mechanisms linking pesticides and

autism," *Environ Health Perspect* 120, no. 7 (2012): 944-951, http://www.ncbi.nlm.nih.gov/pmc/articles/PMC3404662/.

35 "New Mount Sinai study shows exposure to certain pesticides impacts child cognitive development," Icawhn School of Medicine at Mount Sinai, http://www.mssm.edu/about-us/news-and-events/new-mount-sinai-study-shows-exposure-to-certain-pesticides-impacts-child-cognitive-development.

36 V. Rauh and others, "Seven-year neurodevelopmental scores and prenatal exposure to chlorpyrifos, a common agricultural pesticide," *Environ Health Perspect* 119, no. 8 (2011): 1196-201.

37 Forman, "Organic Foods."

38 "USDA Releases 2010 Annual Summary for Pesticide Data Program Report confirms that U.S. food does not pose a safety concern based upon pesticide residues," United States Department of Agriculture, Agricultural Marketing Service, accessed March 20, 2013, http://www.ams.usda.gov/AMSv1.0/.

39 J. P. Reganold and others, "Fruit and Soil Quality of Organic and Conventional Strawberry Agroecosystems," *PLoS ONE* 5, no. 9 (2010): e12346. doi: 10.1371/journal.pone.0012346.

40 S. Y. Wang and others, "Fruit quality, antioxidant capacity, and flavonoid content of organically and conventially grown blueberries," *J Agric Food Chem* 56, no. 14 (2008): 5788-94.

41 "Organic Foods: Health and Environmental Advantages and Disadvantages," accessed March 20, 2013, pediatrics.aappublications.org/content/early/2012/10/15/peds.2012-2579.

42 "Fiscal Year 2009 and 2008 Financial Statements for the Pesticides Reregistration and Expedited Processing Fund," U.S. Environmental Protection Agency Office of Inspector General, accessed March 20, 2013, http://www.epa.gov/oig/reports/2010/20100330-10-1-0087.pdf.

43 "Organophosphate Pesticides," Public Broadcasting Service, accessed March 20, 2013, http://www.pbs.org/tradesecrets/problem/popup_group_05.html.

44 "Smarter Living: Chemical Index," Natural Resources Defence Council, accessed March 20, 2013, http://www.nrdc.org/living/chemicalindex/chlorpyrifos.asp.

45 "Diazinon: Phase Out of all Residential Uses of the Insecticide," U.S. Environmental Protection Agency, accessed March 20, 2013, http://www.epa.gov/opp00001/factsheets/chemicals/diazinon-factsheet.htm.

46 "Carbofuran Cancellation Process," U.S. Environmental Protection Agency, accessed March 20, 2013, http://www.epa.gov/oppsrrd1/reregistration/carbofuran/carbofuran_noic.htm.

47 "Soybeans," Spectrum Commodities, http://www.spectrumcommodities.com/education/commodity/s.html.

48 Anthony Gucciardi, "Monsanto's Roundup spawns superweeds consuming over 120 million hectares," *Natural Society*, November 30, 2011, http://naturalsociety.com/monsantos-roundup-superweeds-consuming-4-million-hectares/.

49 Brian Clark, "Herbicide-resistant crops: more weed resistance means more pesticide used," *WSU News*, October 2, 2012, http://wsunews.wsu.edu/pages/publications.asp?Action=Detail&PublicationID=33169.

50 Rick A. Relyea, "The impact of insecticides and herbicides on the biodiversity and productivity of aquatic communities," *Ecological Applications* 15, no. 2 (2005): 618-627, http://people.sc.fsu.edu/~pbeerli/conservation-bio/web-content/restricted/papers/relyea-2005.pdf.

51 Alejandra Paganelli and others, "Glyphosate-based herbicides produce teratogenic effects on vertebrates by impairing retinoic acid signaling," *Chem. Res. Toxicol.* 23 (2010): 1586-1595, http://big.assets.huffingtonpost.com/carrasco_0.pdf.

52 Caroline Cox and Michael Surgan, "Unidentified inert ingredients in pesticides: implications for human and environmental health," *Environ Health Perspect* 114, no. 12 (2006): 1803-1806, http://www.ncbi.nlm.nih.gov/pmc/articles/PMC1764160/.

53 "Gene Flow and Hybridization Between Jointed Goatgrass and Wheat," United States Department of Agriculture, National Institute of Food and

Agriculture, accessed March 20, 2013, cris.csrees.usda.gov/cgi-bin/
starfinder/0?path=fastlink1.txt&id=anon&pass=&search=AN=0186570
&format=WEBFULL.

54   "Toxic pollen from widely planted, genetically modified corn can kill
monarch butterflies, Cornell study shows," *Cornell News*, May 19, 1999,
http://www.news.cornell.edu/releases/May99/Butterflies.bpf.html.

55   Pew Initiative on Food and Biotechnology, "Three years later: genetically
engineered corn and the monarch butterfly controversy," http://www.
pewtrusts.org/uploadedFiles/wwwpewtrustsorg/Reports/Food_and_
Biotechnology/vf_biotech_monarch.pdf.

56   "History of Agricultural Price-Support and Adjustment Programs,
1933–84," USDA Economic Research Service, accessed March 20, 2013,
ers.usda.gov/publications/aib485/aib485.pdf.

57   "Agricultural policies versus health policies," *PCRM*, http://www.pcrm.
org/search/?cid=2466.

58   Paul C. Westcott, "Ethanol Expansion in the Unites States: How Will the
Agricultural Sector Adjust?" USDA Economic Research Service, http://
www.ers.usda.gov/media/197250/fds07d01_1_.pdf.

59   Susan S. Lang, "Organic farming produces same corn and soybean
yields as conventional farms, but consumes less energy and no pesticides, study finds," *Cornell News*, July 13, 2005, http://www.news.cornell.
edu/stories/july05/organic.farm.vs.other.ssl.html.

60   Rodale Institute, *The Farming Systems Trial*,
http://66.147.244.123/~rodalein/wp-content/uploads/2012/12/
FSTbookletFINAL.pdf.

61   Union of Concerned Scientists, *Cream of the Crop: the economic benefits
of organic dairy farms,* http://www.ucsusa.org/assets/documents/food_
and_agriculture/cream-of-the-crop-report.pdf.

62   Liz Morrison, "Organic Opportunities," *Corn and Soybean Digest,*
January 1, 2010, http://cornandsoybeandigest.com/conservation/
organic-opportunities?page=2.

63 "Organic Corn Profile," Agricultural Marketing Resource Center, accessed March 20, 2013, www.agmrc.org/commodities__products/ grains__oilseeds/corn_grain/organic-corn-profile/.

64 "Economic Data," U.S. Poultry & Egg Association, accessed March 20, 2013, www.uspoultry.org/economic_data/.

65 Environmental Defense Fund, *Resistant bugs and antibiotic drugs: state and county estimates of antibiotics in agricultural feed and animal waste*, http://www.edf.org/sites/default/files/4301_AgEstimates.pdf.

66 Thomas Lund Sørensen and others, "Transient intestinal carriage after ingestion of antibiotic-resistant Enterococcus faecium from chicken and pork," *N Engl J Med* 345 (2001): 1161-1166, doi 10.1056/ NEJMoa010692.

67 Amy R. Sapkota and others, "Arsenic Resistance in Campylobacter spp. Isolated from Retail Poultry Products," *AEM* 72, no. 4 (2006): 3069– 3071, doi: 10.1128/AEM.72.4.3069–3071.2006.

68 *Penn State University News*, "Research shows eggs from pastured chickens may be more nutritious," July 10, 2010. http://live.psu.edu/ story/47514.

69 "Pastured Chickens," Local Harvest, http://www.localharvest.org/ organic-chicken.jsp.

70 "Organic Egg Report and Scorecard," The Cornucopia Institute, http:// www.cornucopia.org/2010/09/organic-egg-report-and-scorecard.

71 Jason Allen and others, "Detoxification in Naturopathic Medicine: A Survey," *Journal of Alternative and Complementary Medicine* 17, no. 12 (December 2011): 1175-1180, http://www.ncbi.nlm.nih.gov/pmc/ articles/PMC3239317.

72 S. J. Padayatty and others, "Vitamin C: Intravenous Use by Complemen- tary and Alternative Medicine Practitioners and Adverse Effects," *PLoS ONE* 5, no. 7 (July 2010), doi: 10.1371/journal.pone.0011414.

73 Qi Chen and others, "Pharmacologic ascorbic acid concentrations selectively kill cancer cells: Action as a pro-drug to deliver hydrogen

peroxide to tissues," *PNAS* 102, no. 38 (September 20, 2005): 13604–13609, doi: 10.1073/pnas.0506390102.

74 L. J. Peng and others, "Therapeutic effect of intravenous high-dose vitamin C on implanten hepatoma in rats," *Nan Fang Yi Ke Da Xue Xue Bao* 29, no. 2 (Feb 2009): 264-266.

75 C. Vollbracht and others, "Intravenous vitamin C administration improves quality of life in breast cancer patients during chemo-/radiotherapy and aftercare: results of a retrospective, multicentre, epidemiological cohort study in Germany, *In Vivo* 25, no. 6 (November-December 2011): 983-90.

76 "Questions and Answers: The NIH Trial of EDTA Chelation Therapy for Coronary Heart Disease," NIH,U.S. Department of Health & Human Services, http://www.nhlbi.nih.gov/news/press-releases/supplement/questions-and-answers-the-nih-trial-of-edta-chelation-therapy-for-coronary-heart-disease.html.

77 Q. Dai and others, "Fruit and vegetable juices and Alzheimer's disease: the Kame Project," *Am J Med.* 119, no. 9 (2006): 751-759.

78 "New Report in Journal of Nutrition, Health and Aging Finds Three Servings Daily Significant," Samueli Institute, www.samueliinstitute.org/about-us/press-room/vegetables-lower-risk-of-dementia.

79 Hsin-Chia Hung and others, "Fruit and vegetable intake and risk of major chronic disease," *J Natl Cancer Inst.* 96, no. 21 (2004): 1577-84.

80 W. G. Christen and others, "Fruit and vegetable intake and the risk of cataract in women," *Am J Clin Nutr* 81, no. 6 (2005): 1417-22.

81 F. J. He and others, "Increased consumption of fruit and vegetables is related to a reduced risk of coronary heart disease: meta-analysis of cohort studies," *J Hum Hypertens* 21, no. 9 (2007): 717-28.

82 "Acupuncture Helps Relieve Chronic Pain," Samueli Institute, www.samueliinstitute.org/about-us/press-room/acupuncture-helps-relieve-chronic-pain.

83 D. Bowden, L. Goddard, and J. Gruzelier, "A randomised controlled single-blind trial of the effects of Reiki and positive imagery on well-being and salivary cortisol," *Brain Res Bull* 81, no. 1 (2010): 66-72. doi: 10.1016/j.brainresbull.2009.10.002.

84 Ellen M. DiNucci, "Energy healing: a complementary treatment for orthopaedic and other conditions," *Orthopedic Nursing Journal* 24, no. 4 (2005): 259-69.

85 M. J. Schlitz and W. G. Braud, "Reiki-plus natural healing: an ethno-graphic/experimental study," *PSI Res* 4, no. 3 (1985): 100–123.

86 A. G. Shore, "Long-term effects of energetic healing on symptoms of psychological depression and self-perceived stress," *Altern Ther Health Med* 10, no. 3 (2004): 42–48.

87 Walter Crinnion, "Components of practical clinical detox programs—sauna as a therapeutic tool," *Altern Ther Health Med* 13, no. 2 (2007): S154-6.

88 Minna L. Hannuksela and Samer Ellahham, "Benefits and risks of sauna bathing," *Am J Med* 110, no. 2 (2001): 118-26.

89 John Paull, "The Future of Organic Agriculture: Otopia or Oblivion?" *Innovative Science Editions* 1 (2010): 11-14, http://orgprints.org/17060/3/17060.pdf.

90 "Making (more) Room for Private Label Organic," Hartman Group, www.hartman-group.com/hartbeat/2007-06-27.

91 John Paull, "The Value of Eco-Labelling: Price Premiums & Consumer Valuations of Organic, Natural, and Place of Origin Food Labels," *VDM Verlag* (2009), http://orgprints.org/16980/1/16980.pdf.

92 "New Zealand Organic Report 2010," Organic-Market.Info.com, www.organic-market.info/web/Continents/Australia-Japan-Pacific/New_Zealand/201/204/0/7914.html.